Low Vision

The Essential Guide for Ophthalmologists

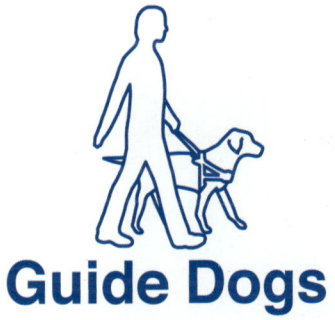

Supported by, designed by and published by
The Guide Dogs for the Blind Association

Published by:

The Guide Dogs for the Blind Association
Hillfields
Burghfield Common
Reading
RG7 3YG

Guide Dogs is a working name of
The Guide Dogs for the Blind Association.

Registered Office: Hillfields, Burghfield Common, Reading, Berkshire, RG7 3YG.
A company limited by guarantee registered in England and Wales (291646) and a charity registered in England and Wales (209617) and Scotland (SC038979).

All rights reserved. No part of this publication may be reproduced, stored in a retrieval system or transmitted, in any form or by any means, electronic, mechanical, photocopying, recording or otherwise, without prior permission of the authors and The Guide Dogs for the Blind Association.

ISBN 978-0-9559268-0-8

Contents

Foreword		**6**
Introduction		**8**
Biographies		**10**
Chapter 1	Definitions, numbers and causes	**12**
Chapter 2	Low vision in daily ophthalmological practice	**20**
Chapter 3	Certification, registration and notification	**32**
Chapter 4	Multi-disciplinary working	**38**
Chapter 5	Magnification and magnifiers	**44**
Chapter 6	Adaptations to daily life	**51**
Chapter 7	Low vision in children	**63**
Poem	Does he have to be so blind?	**74**
Index		**75**

Foreword

People who have suffered permanent loss of vision as adults often have a very clear memory of the consultation at which it was first explained that their eye problem would become a permanent part of their life. Hearing these people tell their story can be a sobering and uncomfortable experience for ophthalmologists, and the task of breaking bad news does not become any easier with experience.

In this beautifully illustrated book, Anne Sinclair and Barbara Ryan equip the ophthalmologist with all the knowledge and practical skills necessary to provide excellent care and advice to patients with low vision and their families. Practical skills such as breaking bad news sensitively, guiding people with severe visual impairment and measurement of visual acuity are explained clearly and simply. Factual information about visual impairment in the UK and the principles of rehabilitation are presented in an interesting and accessible way. It is detailed and well-referenced, yet an enjoyable read from cover to cover.

Ophthalmologists in training will find this book an invaluable resource, both in preparing for examinations and for 'learning on the job'. For the experienced ophthalmologist and other members of the clinical team it will also provide practical ideas for improving services. In short, this book is a 'must read' for all professionals who take part in the care of patients with visual impairments.

I am grateful to the authors for the opportunity to introduce the book, and to The Guide Dogs for the Blind Association for funding its publication.

Brenda Billington

President, the Royal College of Ophthalmologists

Guide dog owners often say that having a dog gives them a new lease of life and an important degree of freedom to go about their daily lives. The journey towards that point, however, can be fraught with difficulties which frequently begin when they are initially diagnosed with a serious sight problem. At this time, confidence can be at a low ebb and depression an ever-present danger.

Indeed, many people report that their loss of confidence around the time of diagnosis prevented them making the progress necessary to maximise their confidence and independence and adapt to their new situation. The good news, though, is that the provision of emotional and practical support at this time can make a very positive difference, helping people find the motivation they need to get on with their lives.

That's why this engaging and attractively designed book will be of such benefit to professionals in the field and, ultimately, to the people who receive their invaluable services. The authors impart their wealth of knowledge with clarity and expertise, providing well-thought out, practical advice to ophthalmologists, backed up with carefully selected information.

We at Guide Dogs are delighted to have been able to assist in the publication of the book and to have had the opportunity to collaborate on its production with the authors and with colleagues in the Royal College of Ophthalmologists. Working together we can truly change things for the better for people with vision loss.

Bridget Warr

Chief Executive,
The Guide Dogs for the Blind Association

Introduction

It is never easy to tell someone that we cannot offer a treatment for their sight loss, or to offer them registration. However, there are many simple strategies that can be incorporated into the way the ophthalmologist practices – even during the busiest clinic – that will ensure the people we encounter experience a smoother journey into accepting their low vision, and living with it.

As professionals who work in the field of low vision, we were delighted that the Royal College of Ophthalmologists recognised the need for training in this area by including it as part of the new curriculum for ophthalmologists in training. This book is designed to support that curriculum.

Anne Sinclair and Barbara Ryan

Barbara would like to thank

Tom Margrain for all his help and support with developing the training modules for optometrists that sparked Anne's idea for this book, and formed the foundation for many of the chapters.

Anne would like to thank
Helen Paterson and Joan Park, her low vision colleagues, for all their help and support.

Barbara and Anne would like to thank:

The Guide Dogs for the Blind Association for funding the book; and the Guide Dogs team – Paul Day, Tom Ferreira, Carl Freeman, Lisa Gillow, Tracey Gurr and Hannah Robertson – for editing, designing and producing the book, and taking most of the photographs.

The Royal College of Ophthalmologists – in particular Brenda Billington, Richard Smith, David Cottrell and Kathy Evans.

Andrew Blaikie and Maggie Woodhouse for their help with the children's chapter.

All the staff at Fife Society for the Blind – but especially rehabilitation worker Anne Williams, social worker Evelyn Hickman and peripatetic teacher Alison Duthie – for their help and advice, and also the volunteers who agreed so willingly to be photographed.

Paul Johnstone and Vikas Chadha for reading through the text from a training viewpoint.

Katie Randerson for public relations and Anne Eadie for promotional materials.

Family, friends and colleagues who have encouraged us to persevere.

Most of all, we would like to thank our patients, from whom we continue to learn.

Biographies

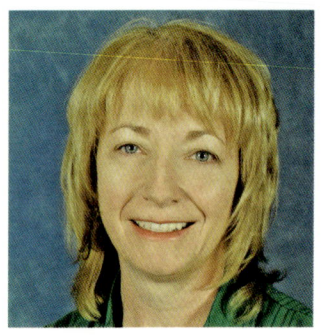

Anne Sinclair is an ophthalmologist in Fife, Scotland, whose main work interest is diabetic eye disease.

Originally from Caithness, Anne studied in Edinburgh before working abroad for ten years, mostly in Africa.

After returning to Scotland, she helped to establish the Fife Interdisciplinary Low Vision Service, where she continues to have one clinic each week alongside a low vision nurse, rehabilitation workers, social workers and visually-impaired volunteers.

Anne has published papers on low vision quality of life, and glaucoma blindness.

She is married to David and has two grown up children, Doug and Jeni.

anne.sinclair@faht.scot.nhs.uk

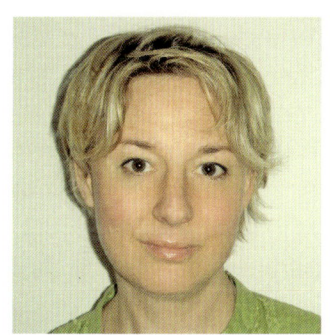

Barbara Ryan is an optometrist based in Wales.

She left her home town, Armagh, in Northern Ireland to study at City University, and then spent her early optometric career in the Hospital Eye Service in Oxford, Birmingham and Nigeria.

In 1995 she started working in the multi-disciplinary Low Vision Team in Birmingham Focus before becoming the first optometrist to work for the national charity RNIB. Barbara's current position at Cardiff University is funded by the Welsh Assembly Government, and includes responsibility for training 160 practitioners who provide the All Wales Low Vision Service.

Barbara's publications on low vision vary from articles in Woman's Own magazine to papers in the British Journal of Ophthalmology.

She continues to practice one day a week in Monmouth, and enjoys living in the Black Mountains with her family Ben, Aran and Charlie.

ryanb@cardiff.ac.uk

1 Low vision: Definitions, numbers and causes

Definitions of low vision

1. **Practical definition for referral to low vision clinic and/or social services.**
2. **WHO (World Health Organisation) definition for research purposes.**

1. Practical definition

Junior ophthalmologists often ask "Which patients should be referred to low vision services?", or "Is there a level of visual acuity below which a patient should be referred?". As in referral for cataract surgery, it depends on the functional vision of the patient, and their visual requirements for daily living.

In the UK, low vision has not been defined in legislation. The definition for low vision adopted by the UK Low Vision Services Consensus Group (which has representation from all relevant professions and organisations) is:

A person with low vision is one who has an impairment of visual function for whom full remediation is not possible by conventional spectacles, contact lenses or medical intervention and which causes restriction in that person's everyday life. This definition includes, but is not limited to, those who are registered as blind and partially-sighted[1].

2. WHO definition

The World Health Organisation defines low vision as:

A visual acuity of less than 6/18, but equal to or better than 3/60 in the better eye with best possible correction[2].

The problem with this definition is that it may exclude many people with a visual impairment whose ability to perform everyday tasks is greatly reduced. For example, someone whose distance visual acuity is 6/12 part would not meet the DVLA's criteria for driving.

Details of the certification and registration processes in use in the UK are outlined in Chapter 3.

The number of people with low vision

Registration data are very useful in considering the extent of low vision in the UK. There are about 346,000 people registered as having a sight problem in Scotland[3], Wales[4] and England[5]. Registration figures may represent an underestimation of the true extent of registrable visual impairment in the population[6]. In addition, many people with a visual impairment do not meet registration criteria but have low vision. The Royal National Institute of Blind People (RNIB) estimates that around two million people in the UK self-define as having a sight problem or seeing difficulty[7].

About 80 per cent of people with a visual impairment are over the age of 65 years[8] (Table 1) and the prevalence increases dramatically with age (Figure 1). As part of the UK-wide Medical Research Council (MRC) trial of assessment and management of older people in the community, Evans et al[9] estimated that there were approximately 609,000 people over the age of 75 years living in the community with visual acuity <6/18 (of which about half had the potentially treatable conditions cataract and refractive error). The prevalence of low vision in the older population is likely to be even higher because this study excluded people in long term nursing care where a higher prevalence has been shown[10]. The magnitude of the problem will undoubtedly grow. Age is known to be a significant risk factor for vision loss[11], and the number of people aged 60 and over is projected to increase by 57 per cent over the next 30 years[12].

Of the 609,000 people with moderate visual impairment in the MRC trial[9], 74 per cent were women. This is not only due to the greater life expectancy of women. It is recognised that women in industrialised countries have an increased risk of visual impairment compared with men[13].

Causes of low vision

The registration process provides a considerable body of data on the causes of visual impairment. Figure 2 shows the causes of certifications for blindness in England and Wales for the year ending March 2000. Data on partial sight registrations for the same year show very similar percentages.

The most common cause of blind (57.2 per cent) and partial sight (56 per cent) certification was 'degeneration of the

Age	0-15	16-64	65-74	75-84	85 and over	Unknown	**Total**
Registered blind	328	1,637	1,692	4,907	4,872	352	**13,788**
Registered partially-sighted	520	2,371	2,855	7,334	5,536	491	**19,107**
Not stated	28	210	202	511	431	133	**1,515**
Total registered	**876**	**4,218**	**4,749**	**12,752**	**10,839**	**976**	**34,410**

Table 1: Numbers of BD8 certificates dated April 1999-March 2000 by visual status in England and Wales[8].

macula and posterior pole' – largely age-related macular degeneration (AMD). Glaucoma and diabetic retinopathy were the next most commonly recorded causes of blind certification.

Of note is the fact that diabetic retinopathy certifications in the over 65 age group more than doubled between the 1990-91 survey and the 1999-2000 comparison. This could be related to the increased prevalence of diabetes, and the longer life expectancy of people who have the disease[14].

The major causes of blindness in the 0 to 15 age group are distinctly different from those in the adult population (Figure 3)[8].

Prenatal factors (including genetic causes) are involved in the majority of cases, and over 40 per cent had either cerebral visual impairment or optic nerve disorders. Over 75 per cent of children with a visual impairment have additional non-ophthalmic disorders or impairments[15].

The ocular complications of diabetes are the most common cause of blindness (Figure 4)[8]. In this age group, the hereditary retinal disorders are also a significant cause of blindness – the most common being retinitis pigmentosa.

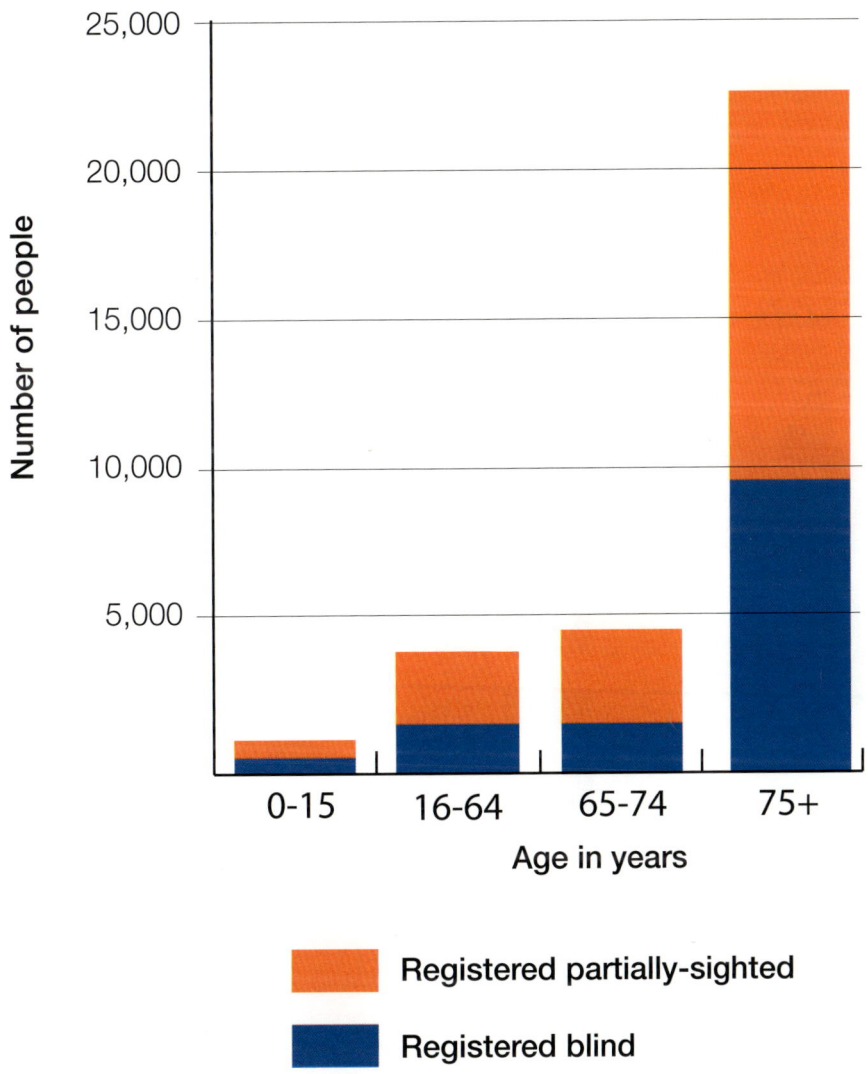

Figure 1: Number of certifications by age in England and Wales, April 1999-March 2000[8].

Chapter 1 Definitions, numbers and causes

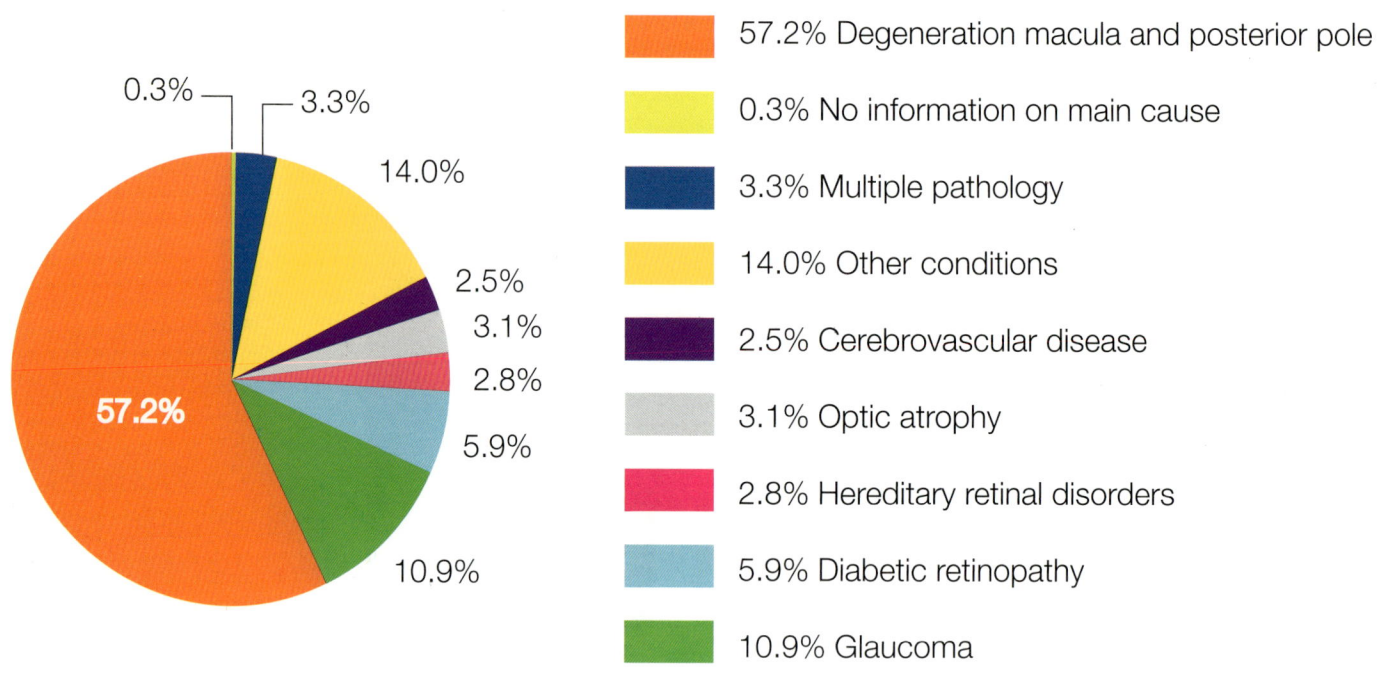

Figure 2: Causes of certifications for blindness in England and Wales, April 1999–March 2000[14].

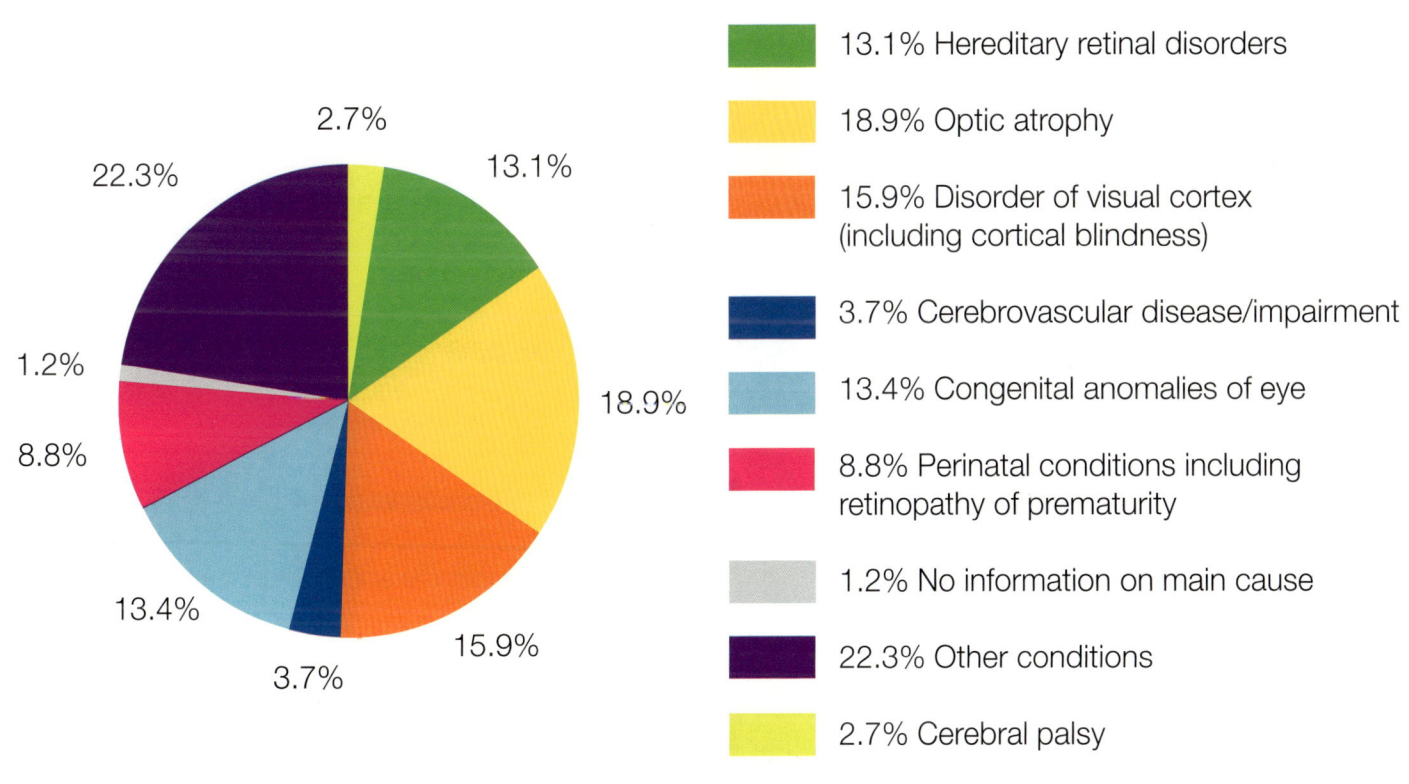

Figure 3: Causes of blindness in England and Wales ages 0–15 years; certifications April 1999–March 2000[8].

Chapter 1 Definitions, numbers and causes

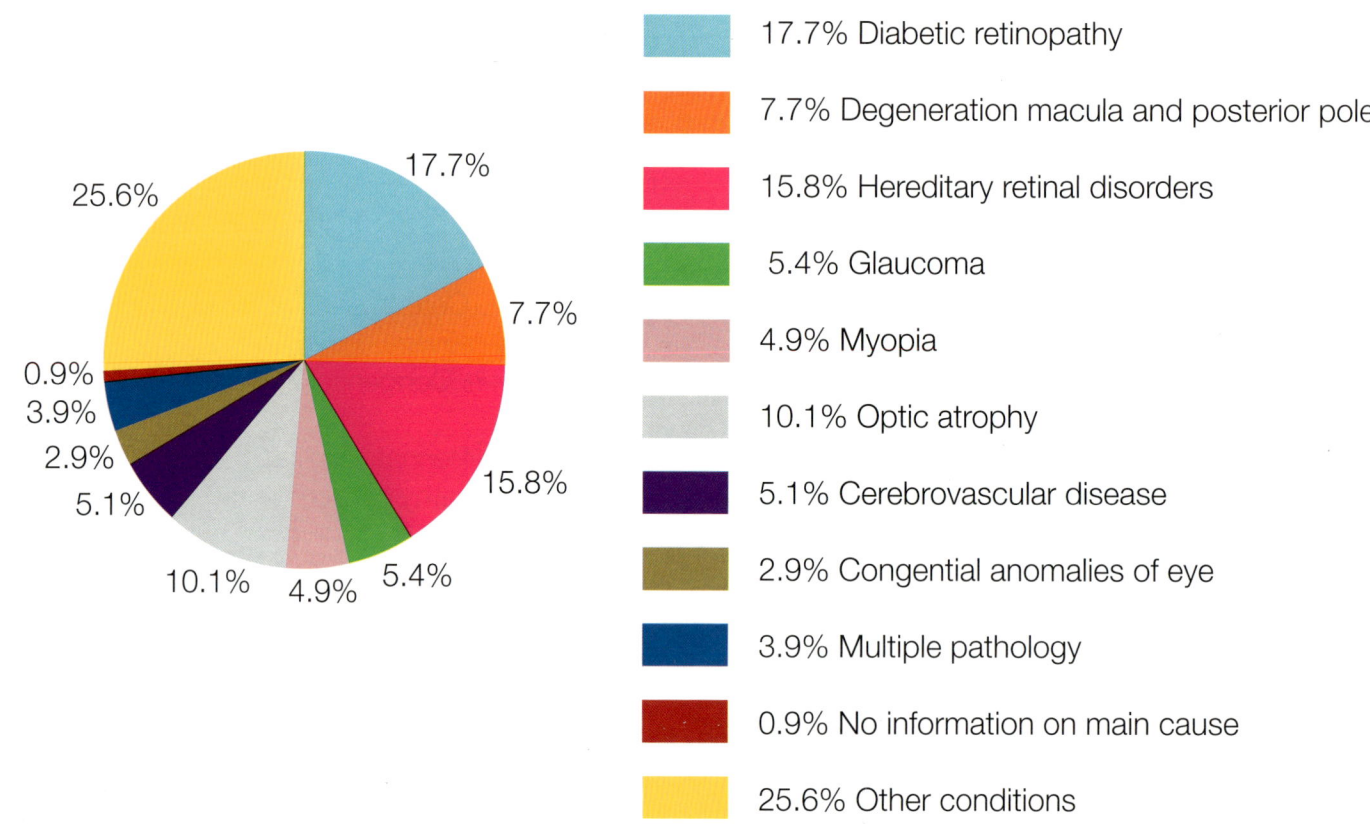

Figure 4: Causes of blindness in England and Wales ages 16-64 years; certifications April 1999–March 2000[8].

References

1. Low Vision Services Consensus Group. Low Vision Services: Recommendations for future service delivery in the UK. London: The Royal National Institute for the Blind, 1999.
2. WHO. The International Classification of Functioning, Disability and Health (ICF). Geneva: World Health Organisation, 2002.
3. Scottish Executive. Registered Blind and Partially-sighted Persons Scotland, 2005.
4. Wales Local Government Data Unit. Register of people with sensory disabilities, 31 March 2006. Cardiff: National Assembly for Wales, 2006.
5. The Information Centre. Registered Blind and Partially-sighted People Year Ending 31 March 2006. London: National Statistics, 2006.
6. Barry RJ, Murray PI. Unregistered visual impairment: is registration a failing system? Br J Ophthalmol 2005;89:995-998.
7. www.rnib.org.uk. Statistics — numbers of people with sight problems in the UK.
8. Bunce C, Wormald R. Causes of blind certifications in England and Wales: April 1999-March 2000. Eye, 2007. (E-published ahead of print)
9. Evans JR, Fletcher AE, Wormald RPL, Ng ESW, Stirling S, Smeeth L, et al. Prevalence of visual impairment in people aged 75 years and older in Britain: results from the MRC trial of assessment and management of older people in the community. Br J Ophthalmol 2002;86:795-800.
10. Van der Pols JC, Bates CJ, McGraw PV, Thompson JR, Reacher M, Prentice A, et al. Visual acuity measurements in a national sample of British elderly people. Br J Ophthalmol 2000;84:165-70.
11. Evans JR, Rooney C, Dettani N, Ashwood F, Wormald RPL. Causes of Blindness and Partial Sight in England and Wales. Health Trends 1996;28:5-12.
12. Shaw C. 2002-based national population projections for the United Kingdom and constituent countries. Population Trends. London: HMSO 2004.
13. Abou-Gareeb I, Lewallen S, Bassett K, Courtright P. Gender and blindness: a meta-analysis of population-based prevalence surveys. Ophthalmic Epidemiology 2001;8:39-56.
14. Bunce C, Wormald R. Leading causes of certification for blindness and partial sight in England & Wales. BMC Public Health 2006;6:58.
15. Rahi JS, Cable N. Severe visual impairment and blindness in children in the UK. Lancet 2003;362:1359-1365.

2 Low vision in daily ophthalmological practice

Although few ophthalmologists participate directly in low vision clinics, they see patients with low vision on a daily basis. People with impaired sight attend eye clinics, whether for their initial diagnosis or for follow up management. A recent survey of patients attending general ophthalmology clinics at Birmingham and Midland Eye Centre found that about 8 per cent had binocular visual acuity of 6/24 or worse[1]. The percentage is likely to be higher in some specialist eye clinics, particularly macular or diabetic eye clinics.

The patient's experience

Visits to eye clinics can be very unpleasant experiences for people who have poor sight[2].

The Royal College of Ophthalmologists (RCOphth) has published guidance for outpatient departments on improving the quality of care to patients. This includes some standards which apply to patients with a visual impairment, such as the print size of appointment letters, signage and visual awareness training for clinic staff[3]. However, many patients still encounter basic difficulties, such as being unable to read clinic appointment letters. When they get to the hospital they may have difficulty reading the signage to clinics. Overcrowded waiting rooms, and poor lighting and contrast add to the stress of the clinic visit, and staff with little awareness of the problems associated with visual impairment may be less than helpful.

So, before the patient has got anywhere near the doctor's consultation room they may have encountered difficulties which have added to the anxiety about their eyesight.

Eventually, it is their turn to see the ophthalmologist. The patient hears their name called from a doorway in the distance, but is unsure where the voice has come from. The doctor thinks he has not been heard and shouts the name louder. There are possibly obstacles on the way – small children with toys, coffee tables, ladies' handbags – and the lighting levels may be far from adequate.

The patient finally reaches the room. The doctor is less than attentive because he is pressed for time. He asks the patient to take a seat but the patient cannot find the chair and is left to fumble around again.

This consultation is off to an unnecessarily bad start. How could it be done better?

Meeting a patient with a visual impairment

1. Check the case notes for an indication of visual acuity before calling the patient.
2. In the waiting room, actively seek the patient out and approach them directly.
3. Introduce yourself and explain where you are going. For example: "I'll take you into the clinic room now."
4. If you think they need help, offer to guide them (see below).
5. On the way, give instructions about where you are going. For example, "my room is the next door on your left" or "the examination chair is a few paces straight ahead of you".

Guiding a patient with a visual impairment

Guiding a person who has a visual impairment (Figure 1) is not difficult, but most people are understandably nervous about offering to guide if they have not had previous experience or training in guiding.

1. Always ask the person if they want help: "Would you like to take my arm?" Never grab their arm and pull them along.
2. When you have established that the patient would like your assistance, give a verbal clue or stand side by side so that the visually-impaired person can locate your upper arm. The person usually then takes a grip just above your elbow.
3. Start moving. You should be about one step ahead of the patient. Never push or drag them.
4. Give commentary concerning any hazards as you walk along. For example, "we are approaching a narrow space" or "we are approaching a flight of stairs going down".
5. If there is not enough room for you to pass through a space side by side, walk in front of the patient so that they can rest a hand on your back.
6. On approaching a door, the patient should be on the hinge side of the door so that they can take control of the door.

Chapter 2 Low vision in daily ophthalmological practice

7. On approaching the examination chair, place a guiding hand on the arm of the chair. The person can then follow your arm down to the arm of the chair and locate the other chair arm before sitting down.

For more detailed instructions on guiding, see the RNIB and Action for Blind People websites[4,5].

History taking

In an ideal world, ophthalmologists would have time to ask patients about the impact their sight loss has on their daily lives, and send detailed referrals to social and rehabilitation services. This is seldom practical in any NHS eye clinic, but the ophthalmologist should at least have sufficient knowledge and understanding of local social and rehabilitation services to be able to offer referral to other professionals according to the needs and wishes of the patient.

A supply of information in accessible formats (for example, tape, CD and large print) is essential, as verbal information is often misinterpreted or forgotten. Where eye clinic liaison workers are employed, this task is much easier.

Taking a comprehensive history from someone with low vision[6] is time-consuming. However, the aim of the ophthalmologist's questions should be to decide whether or not onward referral is required. In a busy clinic, a few open questions such as "how is your sight problem affecting your daily life?" and, if necessary, a few direct questions on the following subjects will give the doctor a quick assessment of the overall situation.

Reading
Most people with low vision will report difficulties with reading. Problems can be experienced with instructions on packets, newspaper print, television listings and computer text. Some people may be happy for others to read their letters and bills for them, but many will wish to do this for themselves. Referral to a low vision clinic for a magnifier may be life changing, and can help people maintain their independence (Figure 2).

Social situation
It is important to know the person's home situation – for example, whether they live alone, have family support or are in sheltered accommodation. An elderly blind patient living alone might require a referral to social services. For those who are particularly vulnerable (for instance at risk

of falling, misuse of medication or suffering burns) a phone call to social services may be required.

Cooking
Those who cook for themselves may not be able to see dials on the cooker or microwave, read recipes, buy food, read instructions on packets, or chop food and pour liquids safely. These issues may be resolved by equipment and training (Figure 3).

Mobility
People with a visual impairment are less likely to go out alone and more likely to have difficulties using public transport[7]. It is easy to lose confidence in crossing roads, for example, and not being able to get out can lead to isolation and loneliness. Orientation and mobility training can often help maintain independence.

Communication
Communication with others also helps to prevent isolation. Large button telephones and free directory enquiry services are helpful. Writing a letter or a list, or just signing one's name, can also pose an enormous obstacle to someone with sight loss. Equipment and training are usually available from rehabilitation services (Figure 4).

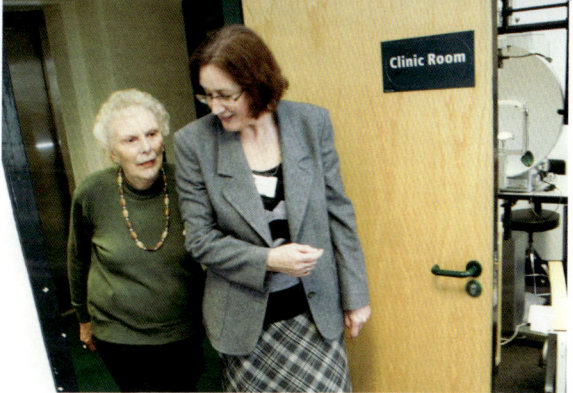

Figure 1: Guiding a patient to your room can be helpful.

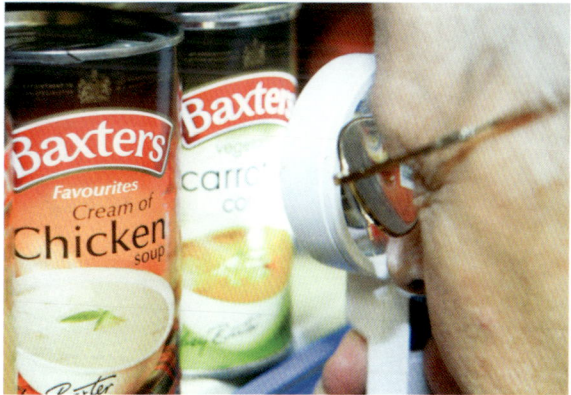

Figure 2: A low vision service may provide a magnifier for shopping.

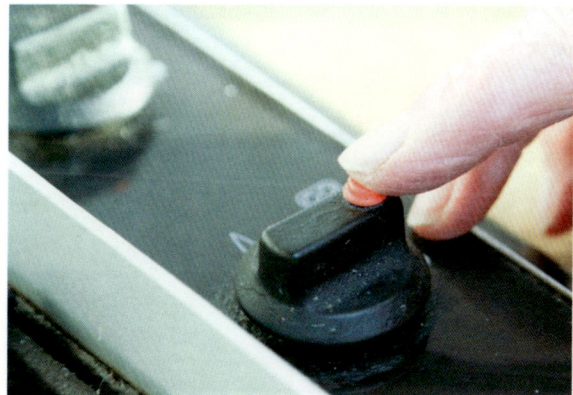

Figure 3: A rehabilitation worker can add tactile markers to appliances.

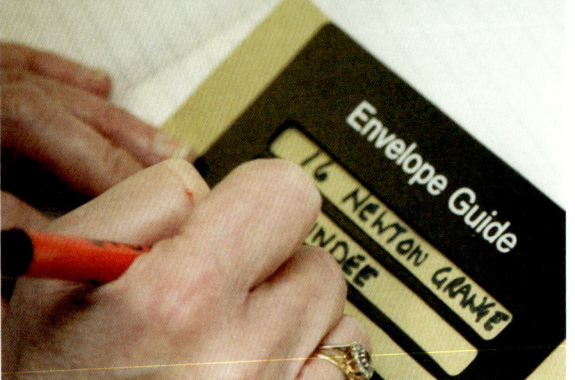

Figure 4: Social services provide equipment and training to aid communication.

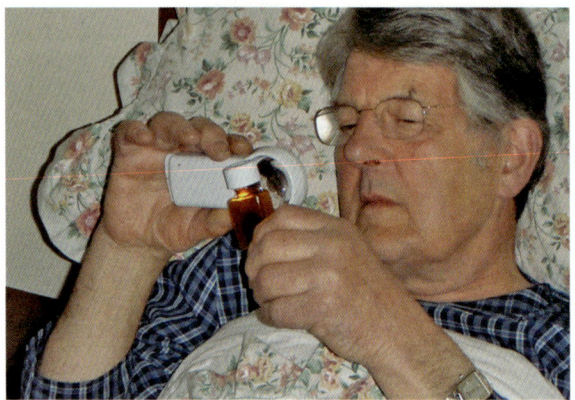

Figure 5: A magnifier makes reading medication instructions easier.

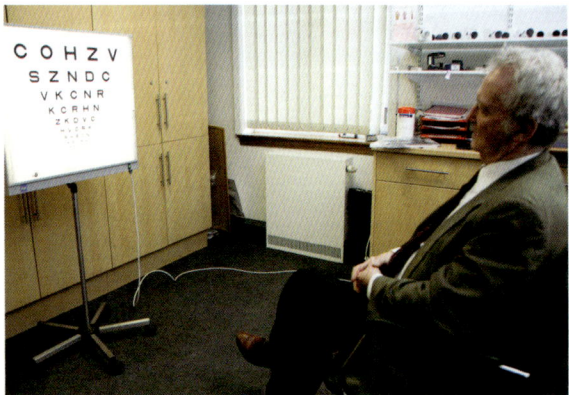

Figure 6: LogMAR charts are preferable to Snellen charts for low vision patients.

Medication
The majority of people with a visual impairment take some form of medication. Determining which tablet to take, measuring injections, instilling eye drops and reading the name and dose can be difficult. A magnifier can help – see Figure 5.

Dual sensory loss
A high proportion of elderly patients with poor sight also have a hearing impairment[8]. The onset of visual problems may make the person more isolated, and lip-reading becomes difficult. It is therefore important to refer such patients to audiology services for a hearing assessment, which is likely to be expedited if dual sensory loss is emphasised by the ophthalmologist.

Glare
Various types of glare are commonly experienced by people with poor vision.
- Disability glare impairs visual function by casting a veil over the retinal image (like turning the lights on in a slide show). Vision is reduced in contrast without necessarily causing discomfort. The person will report seeing better on a dull day.
- Discomfort glare does not necessarily impair visual function.
- Photophobia causes intense discomfort and affects visual function.

Light and dark adaptation

People with low vision, especially those with age-related macular degeneration (AMD), may have a much slower adaptation to increases in ambient illumination. It can take several minutes for vision to be optimised. Patients with retinitis pigmentosa (RP) or end-stage glaucoma may have slow light and dark adaptation. Assessment of home lighting is an invaluable part of the rehabilitation worker's role.

Charles Bonnet Syndrome

A significant proportion of visually-impaired people suffer visual hallucinations, and it is important to remember to ask patients if they ever "see things that are not really there", especially as many will not have told anyone about this. They are usually reassured to hear that it is a very common phenomenon called Charles Bonnet Syndrome[9].

Assessment of visual function

People with poor vision can feel upset or even humiliated by the way in which visual acuity is tested at an eye clinic[2]. Comments such as "you mean you can't see even the big letter at the top?" are very unhelpful. For an accurate assessment, it is important to adapt assessment techniques appropriately, giving the person sufficient time to respond.

Distance visual acuity

The distance visual acuity chart should be placed sufficiently close for the patient to read a line or two of letters. At a functional level, there is a huge difference between a vision of 1.0(6/60) and 'hand movements'. Care should be taken to obtain an accurate assessment between these levels by holding the chart at closer distances if necessary.

Traditional Snellen charts are not recommended for assessing low vision patients, because there are very few letters at poorer acuity levels and increments between lines are largest at poorer levels of acuity. Letters on lower lines are also more 'crowded' than those at the top, causing a variation in the task difficulty.

LogMAR Distance Visual Acuity Charts (Figure 6) are very much more useful within the low vision context[10]. Every row has five letters, which is psychologically better for people with poor acuity as they will probably be able to read five letters if the chart is brought sufficiently close. The separation between each letter and each row is standardised and related to the size of letters. There

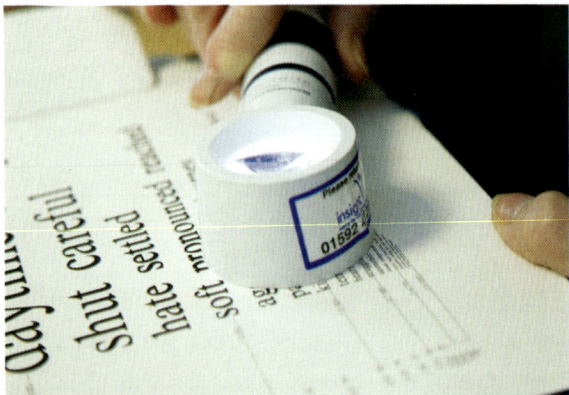

Figure 7: A Bailey-Lovie near test chart.

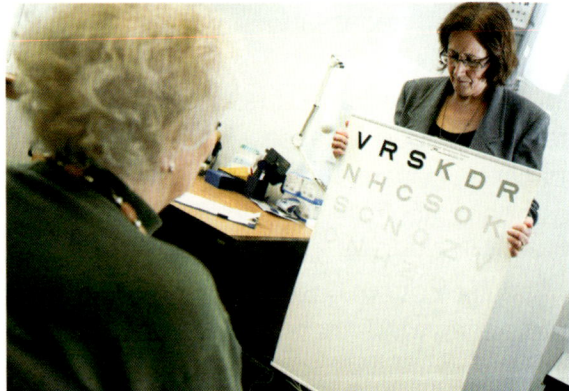

Figure 8: Pelli-Robson chart.

is no variation in 'crowding' and results are legitimate at any distance. There is also uniform progression of letter sizes, increasing in a constant ratio of x1.25 or 0.1 log unit steps.

Near visual acuity

Traditional near charts do not have sufficiently large text for many low vision patients. Near acuity threshold charts have been developed with the needs of the low vision patient in mind. For example, the Bailey-Lovie near chart[11] (Figure 7) incorporates print from N80 to N2.5.

Contrast sensitivity

Contrast sensitivity has found an increasingly important place in visual assessment of people with low vision. The Pelli-Robson letter chart (Figure 8) is easily understood and produces clinical results which are easy to interpret[12]. The chart has letters of a fixed size and is held at a viewing distance of one metre. The contrast of triplets of letters reduces so that a value for the threshold contrast is obtained[13].

Loss of contrast sensitivity causes difficulties in many areas of daily life, from distinguishing money to seeing food on a plate. Reduced contrast affects visually-impaired readers far more than normally sighted people[14]. The inability to see an approaching car, find a door in a room or locate the position of a chair affects outdoor and indoor mobility. Reduced contrast sensitivity has been found to be one of the most significant visual factors in older people falling[15]. Informing rehabilitation professionals that a patient's contrast sensitivity is reduced is important, as improving contrast and lighting can make a significant difference (Table 1) (see Chapter 6).

Visual fields

Visual field testing in a patient with low vision can provide an understanding of functional visual problems. For example, orientation and mobility is most affected by overall constrictions to the visual field or by inferior or central scotomas[17];

Level of function	Contrast threshold	Chart letters		Contrast threshold
Severe loss	99%	VRS	KDR	63%
consider non-sighted techniques	44%	NHC	SOK	31%
Significant loss	22%	SCN	OZV	15%
requires contrast enhancement	11%	CNH	ZOK	7.8%
Noticeable loss	5.6%	NOD	VHR	3.9%
may benefit from improved lighting	2.8%	CDN	ZSV	1.9%
Normal	1.4%	KCH	ODK	1.0%
	0.7%	RSV	HVR	0.5%

Table 1: Pelli-Robson chart contrast threshold values, adapted from Rumney[16].

hemianopias and central scotomas interfere with reading tasks.

In assessing visual fields where the visual acuity is poor the fixation target should be adapted to improve its visibility, and fixation monitoring is usually best turned off. Binocular fields may be adequate and confrontation fields will give sufficient information in many cases. If the patient is being referred for a mobility assessment and training, a copy of the field plot should be made available to their rehabilitation worker.

Amsler grid

Amsler grid testing can give useful information in a small number of patients who are able to describe the size and location of a central scotoma or distortion. An Amsler chart with intersecting lines that form a cross at the centre may help those with central scotomas to maintain fixation. However, Amsler testing is very unreliable, and when a scanning laser ophthalmoscope was used as comparison, the Amsler grid was shown to miss almost half of all scotomas[18].

Breaking bad news

Once the ophthalmologist has examined the patient, determined a diagnosis and decided on a course of action, there can be a tendency and a pressure to attend to the medical aspects of sight loss whilst assuming that 'others' – such as family and friends – will attend to the rest. But it is important to understand that the way the news of sight loss is broken or confirmed can have a huge impact on the person, and remains an enduring memory for each individual[19,20].

All too many people recall the way they were told about their eye condition with anger or disbelief[2]. A rushed or matter-of-fact explanation of a diagnosis can mean that the person spends months or years without knowing the name of their eye condition, or the prognosis.

This may in part be because the patient is not able to take it in. More often it is because a diagnosis has been delivered without sufficient information about the eye condition or about the support that is available.

Breaking bad news 'well'

So what is important when explaining, updating or confirming a diagnosis with a patient? The key points can be summarised as follows:

- Invite the patient to bring a relative or friend into the room if they would like someone else to hear the information you are about to give concerning their eye condition.
- Take the time to sit down with the patient and explain the facts in a clear supportive way, as if you are not in a hurry.
- Give the name of the condition; explain what it is and how it will affect the patient's sight. Give them a leaflet about the eye condition. If this is not possible, at least write down the name of the condition for them.
- Explain that help is available to enable them to make the most of their remaining sight, and provide a signpost to someone who can give more information. For example, this might be their local social services department, a local society or a national organisation such as RNIB or the Macular Disease Society.
- If appropriate, bring up the subject of registration and what it means.
- Acknowledge that you have given them a lot of information to take in, and ask the person if they have any questions.
- If the patient is obviously upset and has no accompanying carer, ask a nurse or other colleague to sit with them and to make sure that they will not leave the building until they have had further support and information.
- When patients have been given bad news, it is essential that they are followed up promptly by social services. Where there are long delays in the referral system, or weak links between health and social services, a review in the eye clinic is indicated.
- When a patient is discharged from the eye clinic they should be made aware of the circumstances under which it would be advisable for them to request a further referral. They must not be made to feel abandoned by the ophthalmologist; especially not with the words "nothing can be done" etched in their memory.

This approach carries a positive message which can make it easier for the patient to seek support from other services.

Psychological factors

Patients react in many different ways to sight loss, and a full discussion of this topic may be found elsewhere[21-24]. In a survey of low vision patients two years after they were registered as blind, the main need they identified was for psychological support – someone to talk to, and an explanation of the pathological condition rather than purely practical assistance[24].

The ophthalmologist should not be expected to act as the patient's counsellor. However, basic counselling skills such as empathic listening and an awareness of the patient's concerns are essential, in keeping with the 'Duties of a Doctor'[25]. The ophthalmologist should not avoid asking the patient how they are coping with their sight loss, and might then, for some patients, suggest referral onwards for counselling or other psychological support as appropriate. Patients who are judged to be clinically depressed should be referred promptly to their general practitioner.

References

1. Barry RJ, Murray PI. Unregistered visual impairment: is registration a failing system? Br J Ophthalmol 2005;89:995-998.
2. Ryan B, McCloughan L. Our better vision: what people need from low vision services in the UK. London: RNIB, 1999.
3. http://www.rcophth.ac.uk/standards. Ophthalmic Services Guidance, Outpatient Department: Royal College of Ophthalmologists, 2006.
4. http://www.rnib.org.uk. How to guide people with sight problems. London: RNIB.
5. http://www.actionforblindpeople.org.uk. Guiding. London.
6. Dickinson C. Low Vision: Principles and Practice. Oxford: Butterworth-Heinemann, 1998.
7. Baker M, Winyard S. Older visually-impaired people in the UK. London: RNIB, 1998.
8. Chia EM, Mitchell P, Rochtchina E, Foran S, Golding M, Wang JJ. Association between vision and hearing impairments and their combined effects on quality of life. Arch Ophthalmol 2006;10:1465-70.
9. Menon GJ, Rahman M, Menon SJ, Dutton GN. Complex visual hallucinations in the visually-impaired: the Charles Bonnet syndrome. Surv of Ophthalmol 2003;48:58-72.

References (continued)

10. Bailey IL, Lovie JE. New design principles for visual acuity letter charts. Am J Optom Physiol Opt 1976;53:740-745.
11. Bailey IL, Lovie JE. The design and use of a new near-vision chart. Am J Optom Physiol Opt 1980;57:378-387.
12. Whittaker SG, Lovie-Kitchin J. Visual requirements for reading. Optom Vis Sci 1993;70:54-65.
13. Pelli DG, Robson JG, Wilkins AJ. The design of a new letter chart for measuring contrast sensitivity. Clin Vis Sci 1988;2:187-199.
14. Crossland MD, Culham LE, Rubin GS. Predicting reading fluency in patients with macular disease. Optom Vis Sci 2005;82:11-17.
15. Lord SR, Dayhew J, Howland A. Multi-focal glasses impair edge-contrast sensitivity and depth perception and increase the risk of falls in older people. J Am Geriatric Soc 2002;50:1760-1766.
16. Rumney NJ. Using visual threshold to establish low vision performance. Ophthal Physiol Opt 1995;15:578-524.
17. Turano KA, Broman AT, Bandeen-Roche K, Munoz B, Rubin GS, West SK. Association of visual field loss and mobility performance in older adults: Salisbury Eye Evaluation. Optom Vis Sci 2004;81:298-307.
18. Schuchard RA. Validity and interpretation of Amsler grid reports. Arch Ophthalmol 1993;111:776-780.
19. Buckman R. How To Break Bad News: A Guide For Health Care Professionals. Basingstoke: Papermac, 1992.
20. Fallowfield L, Jenkins V. Communicating sad, bad, and difficult news in medicine. Lancet 2004 9405:312-319.
21. Faye E. Clinical Low Vision. Boston: Little, Brown and Company, 1984.
22. Crossland MD, Culham LE. Psychological aspects of visual impairment. Optometry in Practice 2000;1:21-26.
23. Williams RA, Brody BL, Thomas RG, Kaplan RM, Brown SI. The psychosocial impact of macular degeneration. Arch Ophthalmol 1998;116:514-520.
24. Conyers MC. Vision for the Future – Meeting the Challenge of Sight Loss. London: Jessica Kingsley Publishers, 1992.
25. http://www.gmc-uk.org/guidance/good_medical_practice/duties_of_a_doctor.asp.

3 Certification, registration and notification

Registration is an important gateway to services and benefits for people with low vision. Although people with sight loss can usually access social services without certification and registration, the process automatically triggers a referral to local support services. Depending on the person's circumstances, registration may also entitle them to financial or other benefits. A list of entitlements is given in Table 1.

The authorities that fund services for visually-impaired people use the epidemiological information gathered during the registration process to help determine the need for services. The World Health Organisation stresses the importance of collecting this data in each country for use in priority setting and resource allocation[1]. Therefore, registering those who are eligible is important to ensure adequate provision of relevant health and social services.

Notwithstanding the importance of the registration process to individuals and to service provision, about half of eligible patients are not registered, despite consultation with an ophthalmologist[2-5]. This may in part be due to lack of awareness on the part of ophthalmologists of all grades, which would benefit from a raised profile for low vision in their training[3]. This is being addressed by the Royal College of Ophthalmologists' new curriculum for specialist training[6].

Consultant ophthalmologists are the only professionals who may complete a certification form on behalf of a patient with visual impairment. The person is then registered by their Local Authority.

Studies conducted in ophthalmology outpatient clinics have shown that a significant proportion of patients with a level of visual impairment that meets the criteria for registration are not certified[2,3,4]. The evidence suggests that those who were excluded from the register saw an ophthalmologist on average four times over a year.

Doctors are more likely to neglect to consider registration for their patients when they are providing treatment for that patient (e.g. in glaucoma or diabetic clinics)[2,3,4], when they are partially-sighted rather than blind[3], and if they are non-white[2,3].

Ophthalmologists in training have a responsibility to alert their consultant to a patient's need for registration. In a busy clinic it can be all too easy to decide that "it can wait until the next review". With emerging therapies for some patients with macular degeneration, there is a danger that they will be sent for urgent investigation and treatment, while their low vision needs are overlooked.

The criteria for registration include both visual acuity and visual field measures. Patients with visual impairment due to visual acuity loss are more likely to be registered than patients with either visual field loss or mixed visual acuity/visual field loss[4]. The ophthalmologist should therefore consider registration in patients with gross peripheral field loss, for example in glaucoma, and not rely simply on the visual acuity criteria.

People may initially be unwilling to be registered because of the stigma attached to being 'blind', or because they are reluctant to be a burden on the state. If not explained carefully, many people reject the process in the first instance. It is vital that discussions are handled in a sensitive manner; encouraging the person by outlining the advantages but allowing them to make the decision for themselves, as it is a voluntary process. Information in an appropriate format, e.g. large print, should be given so that the patient can reconsider their decision after further discussion with family or friends.

The process

The process of registration is currently undergoing change.

In Scotland

For a person to be entered onto the register as 'partially-sighted' or 'blind', their visual impairment must be certified by a consultant ophthalmologist using the form BP1. This has sections to complete concerning the person's demographic details, level of vision, diagnosis, general health, social circumstances and the person's consent to be registered. Once the form has been completed the person is certified as partially-sighted or blind. It is then sent to the local social services department, at which point the person has been registered. In Scotland this system is currently under review.

In Northern Ireland, England and Wales

A new process for registration is now in place. The person is certified by their consultant using a Certificate of Visual Impairment (CVI). The CVI has replaced the BD8 in England and Wales, and the AP655 in Northern Ireland.

There are three parts to the form, and a consent form. The first part contains demographic details and requires the patient's signed consent to be registered. In Part 2 the consultant ophthalmologist records a diagnosis of the condition and information about the person's level of vision. The third part can be filled in by another member of staff in the hospital department, and includes details of the person's living conditions and any other disabilities.

The Local Authority places the person's name on the register and passes the information to the specialist social services, who arrange to carry out an assessment of the person's needs. At this point the person has been registered.

A copy of pages 1-5 of the CVI is sent by the ophthalmologist to the Royal College of Ophthalmologists for the collection and analysis of anonymised epidemiological data. Copies of the new form and guidance notes can be viewed on the Department of Health's website (http://www.dh.gov.uk/assetRoot/04/11/86/66/04118666.pdf).

Along with the CVI, two additional processes with associated forms have been introduced to speed up the provision of services to people with a visual impairment:

- **Optometrist Identification of a Person with Sight Problems – Low Vision Leaflet (LVL).** The Low Vision Leaflet (LVL) is given by an optometrist to anyone with a sight impairment who would benefit from advice and support from social services. It replaces the LVI, which was introduced in England in 2003. The leaflet contains contact details for sources of information, advice and help, both locally and nationally. It also has a short tear-off form with questions for the person to answer about their home situation, difficulties and additional disabilities. If the person completes the form they can post it to their nearest social services department to ask for an assessment. The Local Authority then has a legal duty to advise the person on the range of services available to people with sight loss, and carry out an assessment of their needs.

- **Referral of Visual Impairment (RVI).** Hospital eye clinic staff, with the consent of the patient, can fill in a Referral of Visual Impairment (RVI). The form notifies social services about the person's situation, requests an assessment of need and states how urgently they think the person requires help.

Driving
Information targeted specifically at those who may have a driving licence has been highlighted, warning drivers of the consequences of driving when vision fails to meet the standard requirements.

Categories of certification

Blind
Defined in the Blind Persons Act 1920[7] and subsequently incorporated into the 1948 National Assistance Act[8], as: "So blind as to be unable to perform any work for which eyesight is essential."

With the implementation of the CVI, the terminology in **England, Wales and Northern Ireland** has also been updated and **blind** has been replaced by the term **severely sight impaired**.

Guidelines for measures of visual function for severely sight impaired (blind):
- Visual acuity < 3/60.
- Visual acuity > 3/60 but < 6/60 with a very contracted field of vision (unless this has been longstanding).
- Visual acuity of better than 6/60 with a very constricted visual field, especially in the lower part of the field (excluding people who suffer from homonymous hemianopia or bi-temporal hemianopia with VA better than 6/18).

Partially-sighted
No definition is given, but subsequent guidelines on the National Assistance Act 1948 define partially-sighted as: "Substantially and permanently handicapped by defective vision caused by congenital defect, illness or injury."

With the implementation of the CVI, the terminology in **England, Wales and Northern Ireland** has also been updated and **partially-sighted** has been replaced by the term **sight impaired**.

Guidelines for measures of visual function for sight impaired (partially-sighted):
- Visual acuity of 3/60 to 6/60 with a full visual field.
- Visual acuity of up to 6/24 with moderate restriction of visual field, media opacities or aphakia.
- 6/18 or better with gross field defect (e.g. hemianopia) or a marked constriction of the field (e.g. retinitis pigmentosa).

Benefit or concession	Partially-sighted or sight impaired	Blind or severely sight impaired
Disability Living Allowance (DLA) or Attendance Allowance (AA)	Yes	Yes
Blind person's personal income tax allowance	N/A	Yes
Additional income support or pension credit	Yes	Yes
Council tax reduction	Yes	Yes
Incapacity benefit	Yes	Yes
NHS sight test	Yes	Yes
Television licence reduction	N/A	Yes
Car parking concessions	Possible	Yes
Access to Work equipment and travel costs	Yes	Yes
Articles for the Blind postage	Yes	Yes
Railcard	Yes	Yes
Local travel schemes	Possible	Possible
Free Directory Enquiries	Yes	Yes
Free telephone installation charge and line rental (not Scotland)	Possible	Yes

Table 1: Some of the benefits and concessions for people registered with sight loss

References

1. Bunce C, Wormald R. Leading causes of certification for blindness and partial sight in England & Wales. BMC Public Health 2006;6:58.
2. Robinson R, Deutsch J, Jones HS, Youngson-Reilly S, Hamlin DM, Dhurjon L, et al. Unrecognised and unregistered visual impairment. Br J Ophthalmol 1994;78:736-40.
3. Barry RJ, Murray PI. Unregistered visual impairment: is registration a failing system? Br J Ophthalmol 2005;89:995-998.
4. King AJW, Reddy A, Thompson JR, Rosenthal AR. The rates of blindness and partial sight registration in glaucoma patients. Eye 2000;14:613-619.
5. Bunce C, Evans J, Fraser S, Wormald R. BD8 certification of visually-impaired people. Br J Ophthalmol 1998;82:72-76.
6. http://curriculum.rcophth.ac.uk/. 2007.
7. The Blind Person's Act London: HMSO, 1920.
8. National Assistance Act. London: HMSO, 1948.

4 Multi-disciplinary working

People with low vision may benefit from input provided by a wide range of services and professionals. In this context, the ophthalmologist is part of a multi-disciplinary team which should assist the person with low vision to stay as autonomous and confident as possible.

The input required from each professional will vary according to the particular needs of individual patients, and a 'one size fits all' approach will fail to address the issues facing each person trying to cope with sight loss. Unlike the traditional view of team-working, the members of this team may never meet. However, the provision of good low vision rehabilitation heavily depends on the ophthalmologist's ability to communicate effectively with the other team members[1]. This is time consuming and often frustrating, but will make a difference to the final outcome for your patients.

Health care services

In the UK, low vision services have been described as 'fragmented and patchy'[2]. This view has been confirmed by two surveys of low vision services[3,4].

Low vision services have traditionally been provided in hospitals by optometrists or dispensing opticians, but also by orthoptists and, occasionally, ophthalmologists[5]. Increasingly, these services are also provided in multi-disciplinary centres or in community optometry practice[6,7].

Low vision service provision offers a range of interventions which aim to minimise disability by making specific tasks easier to perform. This is achieved by helping people to make full use of the sight they have by providing equipment, training and advice.

It is essential that ophthalmologists familiarise themselves with their local low vision services, and how to refer patients appropriately to those services.

Social services

People with poor vision have a right to social services because they fall within the definition of 'disabled' as outlined in the Community Care Act 1990[8]. There is therefore an obligation for the Local Authority to assess the needs of a person with sight loss and then provide a package of measures addressing their psychological, social, physical, financial, practical and environmental needs.

Some of the services may be provided by external agencies or the voluntary sector on a contracted basis. There may be many different professionals within a social services department who are called upon to form this package of services, but usually they will be social workers and rehabilitation workers.

Social workers

Social workers are now educated to degree standard, through a course which incorporates practice-based study. Social workers will undertake an assessment of need, and arrange support services. Emotional support may also be provided where appropriate. Some areas have social workers who specialise in working with people with a visual impairment, and who work within multi-disciplinary teams alongside rehabilitation workers. Social workers are generally employed by Local Authority social services, although some work in local voluntary organisations and hospitals.

Rehabilitation workers

The qualification required to practice as a rehabilitation worker is a Diploma of Higher Education in Rehabilitation Studies, or the new BSc (Hons) in Healthcare Practice (Rehabilitation of Visual Impairment).

Rehabilitation workers are trained to work with the person in their own environment, and provide practical solutions to overcome the difficulties resulting from visual impairment. Their training includes knowledge of common eye diseases and an understanding of the consequent functional problems.

Rehabilitation workers are employed by social services departments, and in some cases by local charities where services have been contracted out. They may work in sensory disability teams alongside social workers and others to provide services to people with hearing and/or visual impairments.

The Community Care process

A Community Care assessment for a visually-impaired person is usually provided by a sensory disability team or a general social services team with a special interest in visual impairment. An assessment is carried out to establish the measures necessary to overcome practical and/or emotional difficulties.

From the information gathered, a care plan is formulated. This outlines the necessary adaptations to the person's home, and the training needs of the person. If the plan is wide ranging a care manager or key worker is appointed to ensure that the care is co-ordinated.

Types of assistance provided:

- Adaptations to the home use the basic low vision concepts of good lighting, contrast enhancement and enlargement. New lighting may be installed, or non-optical low vision aids such as coloured chopping boards or large number watches may be recommended. Adaptations for the use of a magnifier may be advised, such as reading stands or task lighting.
- Daily living skills help people with low vision manage the tasks they need to do around the home by maintaining confidence and independence. A rehabilitation worker identifies problem areas and develops a rehabilitation training programme. This may include kitchen skills, personal care and general household tasks, including the use of low vision aids as appropriate.
- Orientation and mobility training may be provided to anyone who has a visual impairment and has difficulty getting about. The assessment and training will take into account the routes the person wants to travel, their level of vision, mobility aids, low vision aids, physical fitness, preparation for a guide dog and use of a sighted guide.
- Many other services may be incorporated into a care plan for someone with a visual impairment. These might include benefits rights, occupational therapy, counselling, day care and Meals on Wheels.

The ophthalmologist's role in relation to social services

Junior ophthalmologists should visit a local social services team and find out how they operate. A home visit with a social worker or rehabilitation worker is an invaluable part of ophthalmology training, and is recommended in the Royal College of Ophthalmologists' Curriculum for Ophthalmic Specialist Training[9].

Once appointed to a consultant post, he/she should again make contact with the relevant local social services professionals, and ensure that good lines of communication are established and maintained. The importance of the ophthalmologist as a fully participating member of the multi-disciplinary team cannot be over-stressed.

Referral prior to the certification process

Patients with sight loss may benefit from social services input before they are eligible for certification. Early referral can relieve anxiety and enable the person to begin to adapt to their changing vision, rather than having to cope alone and unsupported until an ophthalmologist notices that their visual acuity has dropped to the level at which they can complete a form on the patient's behalf.

Ophthalmology departments should have established lines of communication with local social services, and be able to contact the relevant professionals about their patients. A referral in writing or by informal telephone message might be useful if:

- A person is not registered but would benefit from social services input.
- An aspect of a person's life has been identified that may lead to them harming themselves or someone else (e.g. danger in the kitchen, or risk of falling).
- The person's situation has changed since social services were last involved, e.g. a spouse has died.

Informed consent from the patient is always necessary before such a referral can be made.

Education services

See Chapter 7.

Employment services

People who have a visual impairment can get help to find or stay in employment through the Access to Work scheme, which operates by giving one-off or ongoing grants to provide:

- Adaptations to equipment or to work premises. This can include provision of CCTVs, software for computers, Braille keyboards and task lights. Job seekers are eligible for a full grant, and those who are employed are eligible for 80 per cent of the cost, with the

remainder being covered by the employer.
- Support workers.
- Travel to and from work.

People of employment age who have a visual impairment and are not aware of the Access to Work scheme should contact their Local Employment Centre (Job Centre). The scheme is administered by the disability service team. A disability employment advisor (DEA) will give advice on eligibility, provide information about the scheme and assist the person in applying. A workplace assessment is then carried out by a technical officer from the Local Employment Centre. In some areas this has been contracted out to other organisations.

Voluntary organisations

These can be divided into four main groups.

1. Disease specific groups provide information and peer support to people who have similar eye conditions. Groups exist for many eye conditions, including macular degeneration, glaucoma, nystagmus, retinitis pigmentosa and diabetic eye disease. All UK groups can be contacted by calling the RNIB Helpline on 0845 766 9999.
2. Hobby-specific groups link people with a visual impairment who have similar interests. They include music groups and sports groups.
3. Voluntary organisations exist in most areas to provide advice and support at a local level. Most run social events and provide or sell adaptive equipment. Some offer extensive services and hold the Local Authority contract to provide rehabilitation services to people with a visual impairment in the area.
4. National organisations such as The Guide Dogs for the Blind Association, The Royal National Institute of Blind People, Action for Blind People and the Partially-sighted Society provide information and advice and campaign on behalf of people with visual impairment.

References

1. Provision of Low Vision Care. London: The Royal College of Ophthalmologists, 1998.
2. Dickinson C. Low vision: a parochial approach. Br J Ophthalmol 1995;79:715-716.
3. McLaughlan B, Lightstone A, Winyard S. A question of independence: A call for action to improve sight loss support services across the UK. London: RNIB, 2006.
4. Ryan B, Culham L. Fragmented Vision. Survey of Low Vision Services in the UK. London: RNIB and Moorfields Eye Hospital, 1999.
5. Culham LE, Ryan B, Jackson AJ, Hill AR, Jones B, Miles C, et al. Low vision services for vision rehabilitation in the United Kingdom. Br J Ophthalmol. 2002;86:743-747.
6. Adams OF. Rehabilitation: a multidisciplinary approach. In: Jackson AJ, Wolffsohn JS, editors. Low Vision Manual. Philadelphia: Butterworth Heinemann Elsevier, 2007.
7. Eye Care Services Steering Group report: Eyecare Pathways: Cataract, glaucoma, AMD, low vision. London: Department of Health, 2007. www.dh.gov.uk/assetRoot/04/08/09/99/04080999.pdf.
8. National Health Service and Community Care Act 1990. London: HMSO.
9. http://curriculum.rcophth.ac.uk/.

5 Magnification and magnifiers

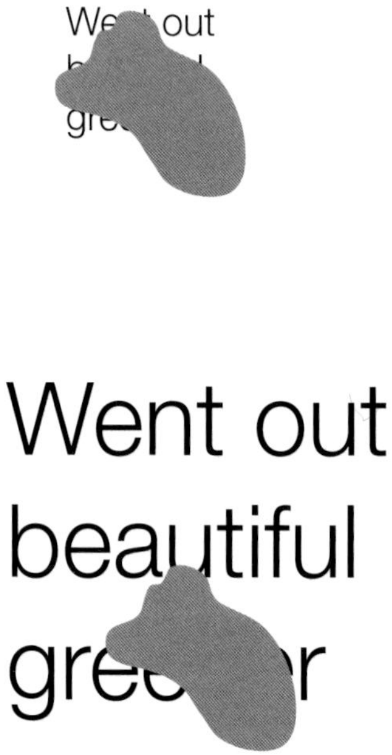

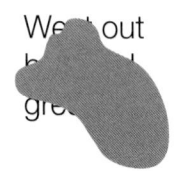

Many people with low vision find magnifiers useful to help them do short everyday tasks such as reading their post or instructions on a packet. Magnification increases the retinal image size. For people with a scotoma this may make an object easier to see, because although the retinal image size increases the area of visual loss remains the same size (Figure 1).

1. Relative size magnification

This is a linear relationship: doubling the size of the object makes the image on the retina twice as large, creating x2 magnification. This form of magnification is usually limited to about 2.5x because of the physical limitations of enlarging an object. Examples of this type of magnification are large print books, watches or timers (Figure 2).

2. Relative distance magnification

This is also a linear relationship: halve the distance of the object and the retinal

Figure 1: A schematic and simplified representation of how magnification can help a person to read short text.

image becomes twice as large, creating x2 magnification. For example, viewing the television from 2m rather than 4m gives x2 magnification (Figure 3).

This type of magnification can also be used for near tasks, e.g. bringing print closer to the eye from 40cm to 10cm gives x4 magnification.

Children and young adults can use accommodation to provide this form of magnification, mainly for short duration near tasks. Myopes who take off their glasses can achieve some magnification without the need for accommodation.

Plus lens magnification

A plus lens creates magnification by allowing the person to adopt a closer viewing distance. When the plus lens is placed so that the object viewed is at the anterior focal point of the lens, the object is focused clearly on the retina and accommodation can be relaxed. Most hand and stand magnifiers work on this very simple principle. The plus lens can be close to the eye, in a spectacle lens, or remote from it, in a hand or stand magnifier.

Limitations of plus lens magnifiers
- Field of view: Patients often ask for larger magnifiers, hoping that this will

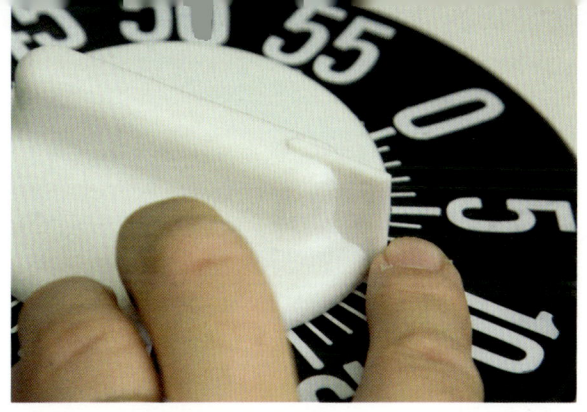

Figure 2: Making things bigger creates relative size magnification.

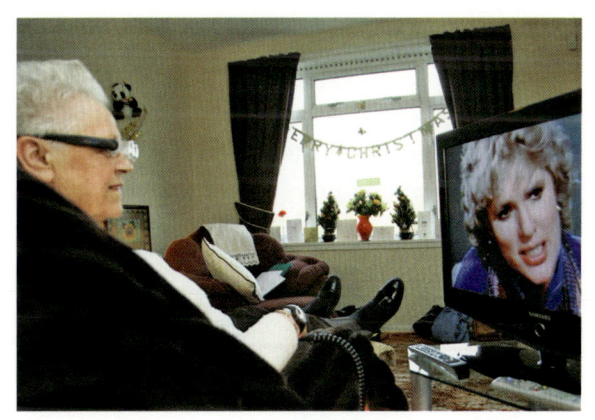

Figure 3: Moving things closer creates relative distance magnification.

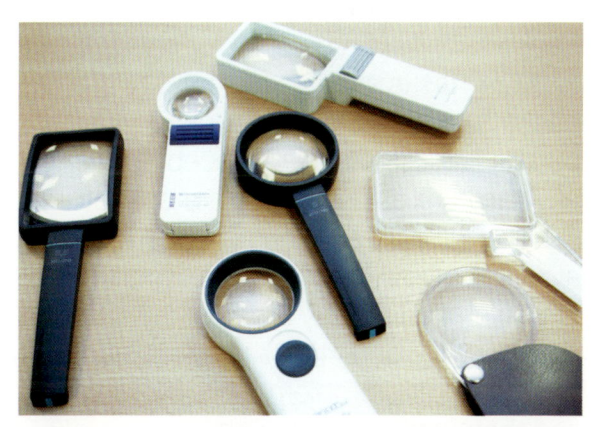

Figure 4: A wide range of hand magnifiers is available, including folding and illuminated versions.

Chapter 5 Magnification and magnifiers 45

increase their field of view. However, as the power of a magnifier increases, the diameter of the lens decreases, due to the weight of the lens and physical constraints in manufacturing. Instead, they should be encouraged to hold the magnifier as close as possible to the eye, thereby increasing the field of view.

- Short working distance: Although the distance from the eye to the magnifier can be varied, the distance from the magnifier to the object is often very short, especially with stronger magnification. This makes it difficult to place implements such as a pen or screwdriver under stronger magnifiers, and directing adequate light on to the object can be problematic.

Hand magnifiers

Hand magnifiers are useful for short 'survival' tasks such as looking at packets or the dials on a cooker. Most people find them socially acceptable and they are easy to carry in a pocket or handbag. There are countless designs available at low cost in a wide range of powers, and many are internally illuminated (Figure 4). People with hand tremors or grip problems may, however, find them impossible to use.

Stand magnifiers

Stand magnifiers allow the maintenance of a precise magnifier-to-object distance, which is advantageous because of the small depth of focus of plus lens magnifiers. This means they are particularly useful for sustained tasks or where there are physical difficulties, such as tremor. The most commonly prescribed stand magnifiers are internally illuminated because the stand can obstruct light from getting to the object (Figure 5). Some lower-powered stand magnifiers allow tools, such as a pen, to be used (Figure 6). The disadvantage is that they are very bulky.

Spectacle-mounted plus lens magnifiers

The best optical solution to the difficulties of plus lens magnifiers is to mount them in spectacles: this gives the best magnification and greatest field of view. However, the majority of patients do not like any magnifier that focuses less than 25cm from the spectacle plane. For people who are able to accept shorter working distances, spectacle-mounted plus lenses are sometimes tolerated because they give the best magnification and field of view, and allow their hands to be free (Figure 7).

Spectacle-mounted low vision aids can be prescribed monocularly or binocularly

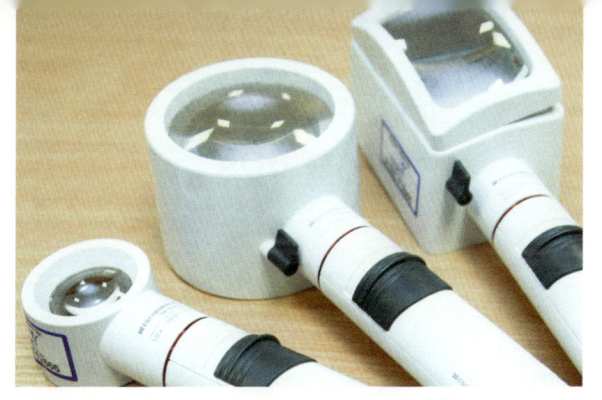

Figure 5: Illuminated stand magnifiers are the most commonly prescribed stand magnifiers.

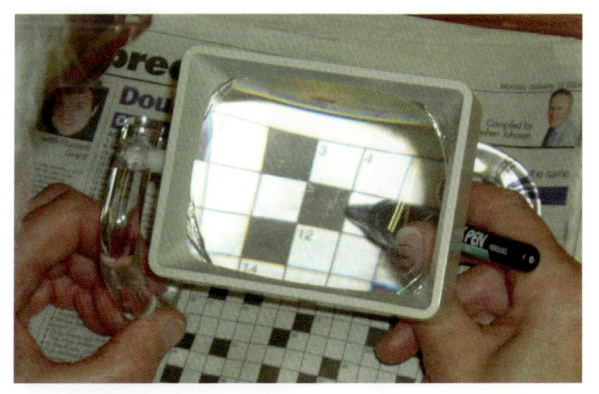

Figure 6: A pen may be used under some low powered stand magnifiers.

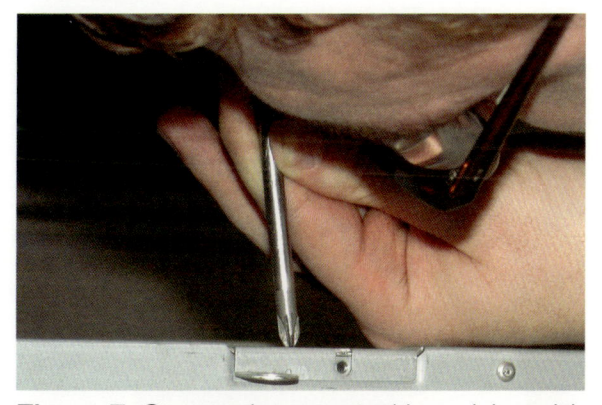

Figure 7: Spectacle-mounted low vision aids allow the person to do tasks that need both hands free, but only at a short working distance.

if prisms are incorporated to help convergence. Over +10.00DS, the person is unlikely to maintain binocularity. As well as providing magnification, some allow for the correction of refractive errors; high powered bifocal near additions are also available.

3. Real image magnification

Optical magnifying systems are limited to a magnification of about x20. Real image magnification produced electronically is available in much larger magnifications of x50 and over.

Closed circuit televisions

Closed circuit televisions (CCTVs) produce real image magnification electronically using a camera to create a magnified image on a monitor screen. They are usually used for near or intermediate tasks.

In theory, CCTVs should be the solution to all the frustrations of low vision aid users. They can produce high degrees of magnification, contrast reversal and enhancement, zoom facilities and binocularity of the image with none of the postural difficulties of many other magnifiers. In practice, however, they are

Chapter 5 Magnification and magnifiers

expensive, quite difficult to use and often bulky. Only a small proportion of the low vision population use CCTVs, and most do so for longer, sustained reading tasks while they use optical low vision aids for short, survival tasks.

The most common type of CCTV is a TV screen mounted above an 'X-Y' table where the object is placed or held (Figure 8). Standard CCTVs cost about £1,500 but many models are much more expensive. TV readers are more affordable (£100 to £500). They consist of a hand-held camera which is plugged into the patient's own television (Figure 9). The magnification is limited, often fixed at one value and dependent on the size of the television screen. Although they are cheap and quite portable, they are difficult to manipulate.

In recent years a number of head mounted CCTVs have been developed, such as the Jordy. The camera and TV screens are mounted in a virtual reality-type headset, and the control box is attached to the belt. These remain very expensive, heavy, difficult to use and cosmetically poor and, as yet, they cannot be used when walking around.

Unlike optical low vision aids, CCTVs are not provided on the NHS. Employment and education services will usually provide

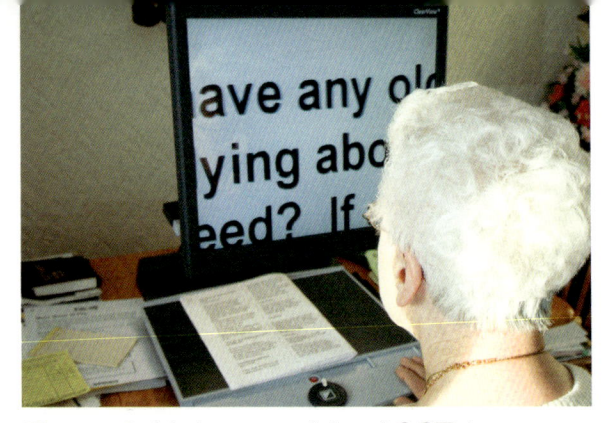

Figure 8: Various models of CCTV are available. The material to be viewed is placed on an X-Y table.

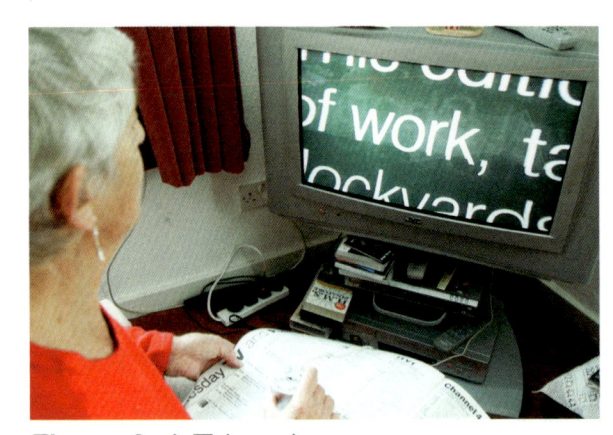

Figure 9: A TV reader.

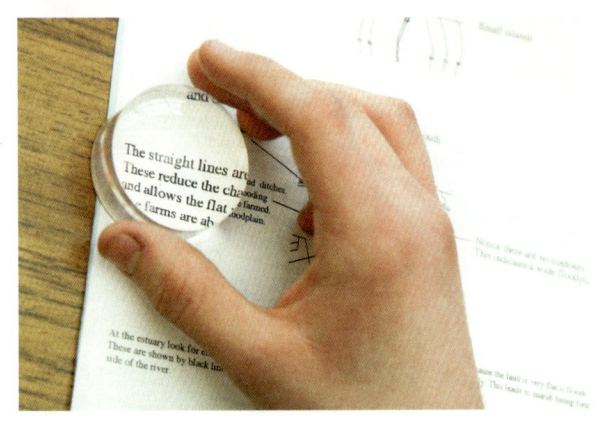

Figure 10: A flat field magnifier.

them if deemed necessary for the person's work or schooling. Older people usually have to purchase their own. Many public libraries, some voluntary organisations for blind people and some social services departments have them available for trial use. Most manufacturing companies will let people try the CCTV in their own home for a short period before purchase. Due to the great expense and difficulty involved in using CCTVs, this approach should be strongly recommended to patients.

Flat field magnifiers
These are single lenses of hemi-cylindrical or hemispherical form, designed to be put flat onto the object (usually text). The thicker the magnifier is in relation to its radius of curvature, the higher its magnification. This is unlikely to exceed x3 because of size and weight. Flat field magnifiers are very useful for children with a visual impairment as they look like a paperweight or 'crystal ball' (Figure 10).

4. Angular (or telescopic) magnification

Telescopes and binoculars are very effective in producing magnification for distance, while allowing the person to stay at their chosen distance from a task, such as viewing a street sign or blackboard. They can also be used for near tasks. Their main disadvantage is restricted field of view. Also, distortion of space and movement perception prohibits walking around while using the telescope. Their use requires considerable manual dexterity, skill and practice, particularly to follow moving objects. Only a very small proportion of people with low vision use them (Figure 11).

Low vision therapy

Although as yet there is no conclusive evidence[1], it is thought that people may benefit from training which maximises the usefulness of low vision aids and vision in daily life. Some rehabilitation workers are trained to provide low vision therapy, which may take place outdoors with distance aids or in the person's home environment.

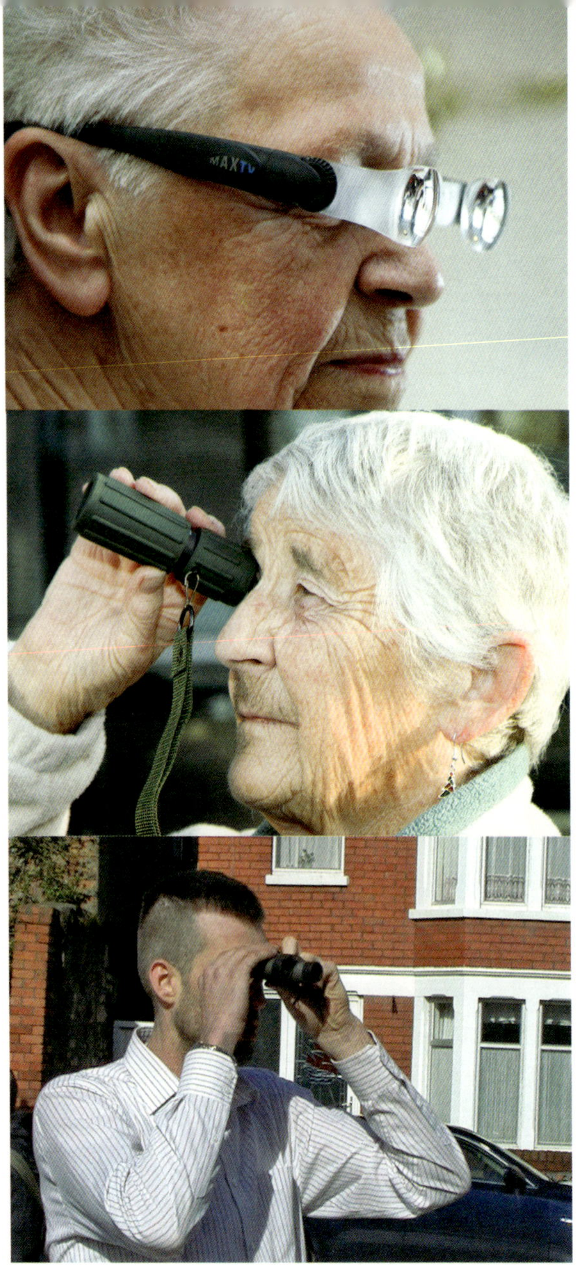

Figure 11: Devices that produce angular magnification: a distance Galilean telescope used for TV viewing, terrestrial telescope and a pair of binoculars.

References

1. Reeves B, Harper R, Russell W. Enhanced low vision rehabilitation for people with age related macular degeneration: a randomised controlled trial. Br J Ophthalmol 2004; 88:1443-1449.

Further reading

Elkington AR, Frank HJ, Greaney MJ. Clinical Optics: Blackwell Science, 1999

Dickinson C. Low Vision Principles and Practice. Oxford: Butterworth-Heinemann, 1998

Jackson AJ, Wolffsohn JS. Low Vision Manual. Philadelphia: Butterworth-Heinemann-Elsevier, 2007

Product Catalogue Associated Optical (Eschenbach and COIL magnifiers)

Product Catalogue Schweizer

Adaptations to daily life

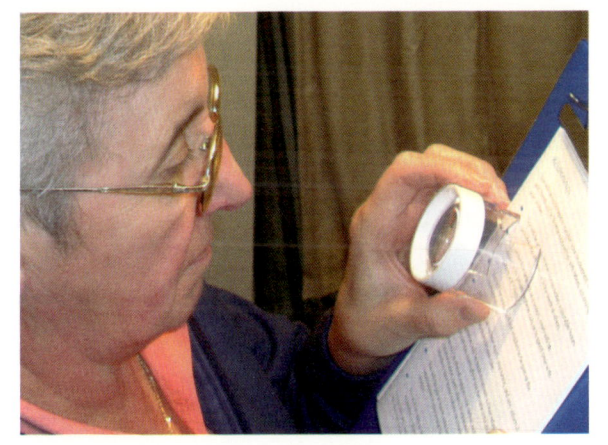

Figure 1: A clipboard allows a person to rest their magnifier on a flimsy page.

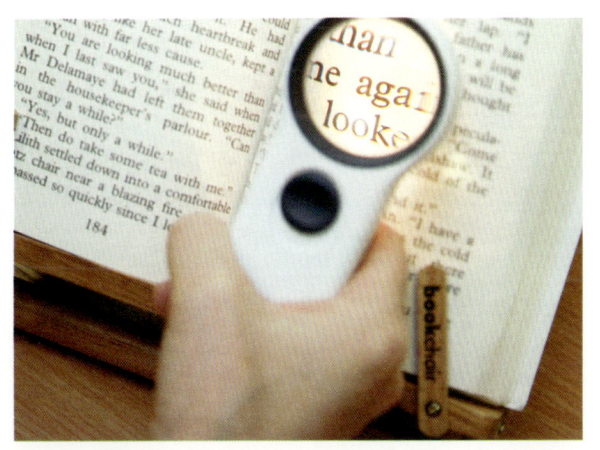

Figure 2: A reading stand allows a more normal posture when using a magnifier.

When ophthalmologists think of low vision aids, an image of a magnifier usually comes to mind. However, there are many devices and strategies that can enable a person with sight loss to use their residual vision and other senses to best advantage.

1. Postural aids

A common reason for not using a prescribed magnifier is that it requires an unnatural and uncomfortable posture. Clipboards and reading stands keep flimsy material flat, encouraging better posture (Figures 1 and 2).

2. Reading techniques

Eccentric viewing
A person who has a central scotoma may benefit from using eccentric viewing (EV), particularly if the scotoma is small. Some patients find their preferred retinal location (PRL) naturally, but others need help. Objects such as a clock may be more

easily seen with the head turned to one side. Moving the eyes rather than the head for non-reading tasks, such as watching TV, can be more comfortable. Using EV to read is more difficult, but studies of intensive training have shown improvements in reading for some patients[1].

Steady eye strategy

It is extremely difficult to read by tracking along a line of print with a magnifier while keeping within a PRL. Some patients with a central scotoma may find it easier to keep their eyes still and use eccentric fixation while moving the text from right to left. This 'steady eye strategy' allows the letters to be imaged in turn on the preferred retinal location. It also has the advantage of enabling the reader to constantly use the centre of the lens, maximising image quality. This is easier with CCTVs than with optical devices[2]. For a more detailed explanation of special reading techniques, see Dickinson[3].

3. Aids for peripheral visual field loss – field expanders

A small proportion of patients with visual field loss and relatively spared central vision, e.g. in retinitis pigmentosa, may benefit from aids for peripheral field loss. However, the majority find them disorientating and difficult to use. Field expanders work on the principle that if a scene is minified then more information is available within the limited remaining visual field.

Such systems include reverse telescopes, hand-held minus lenses, mirror spectacles and prismatic systems[3]. With all field expanders, a person's visual acuity is reduced and perception of depth and movement is distorted. For this reason they are used mainly for the static location of objects.

4. Mobility aids

A mobility aid assists a person with navigating safely and comfortably from place to place. A sighted person guiding a person with a visual impairment (sighted guide technique) is one method of achieving this[4] (see Chapter 2).

Guide dogs

Only a very small number of people with a visual impairment use guide dogs (Figure 3). People with severe sight loss can self-refer for assessment with The Guide Dogs for the Blind Association[5], or may be referred by a social worker,

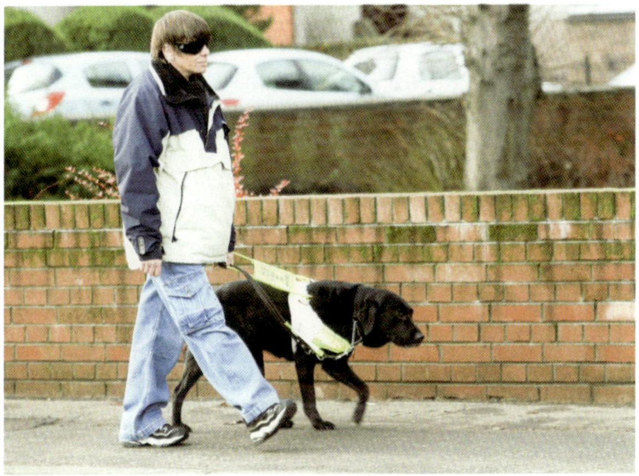

Figure 3: A guide dog assists with crossing roads and avoiding obstructions.

rehabilitation worker, general practitioner or ophthalmologist. A guide dog owner must be over 16, and needs to be fit and active enough to walk and care for a dog. Applicants receive extensive training with the dog. The owner must be able to direct the dog as to a given route.

White sticks and canes

There are four types of white stick or cane (Figure 4):
- A symbol cane is made from sections of folding lightweight tube. It is designed to indicate that the user has a visual impairment, e.g. in a busy shopping street. The user should have some training in its use. Symbol canes are available from social services and voluntary agencies.
- The guide cane is longer and sturdier than the symbol cane, and is used by people with some vision to identify kerbs, steps and stairs. It must be issued by a rehabilitation worker as instruction and training are required.
- A long cane is a long, lightweight cane with a rubber grip and a roller ball tip. It is used by people who have very little vision to scan the ground ahead and identify obstacles or hazards. Again, a course of instruction is needed.
- A white walking stick is used by people who need support for walking, and generally acts as a symbol rather than navigation aid. Occupational therapists or physiotherapists usually prescribe these.

Figure 4: There are four main types of stick that people with a visual impairment use:

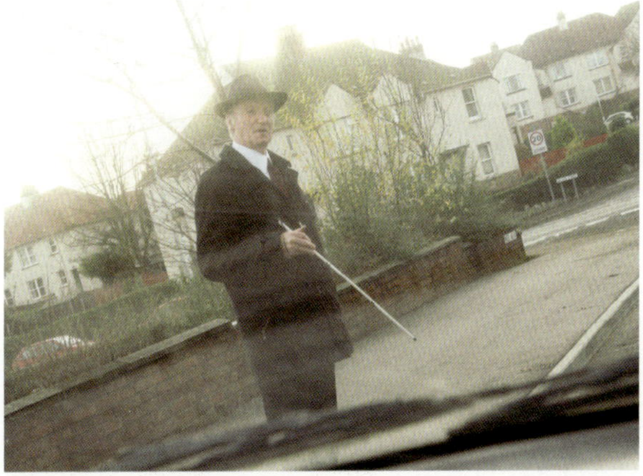

Symbol cane.

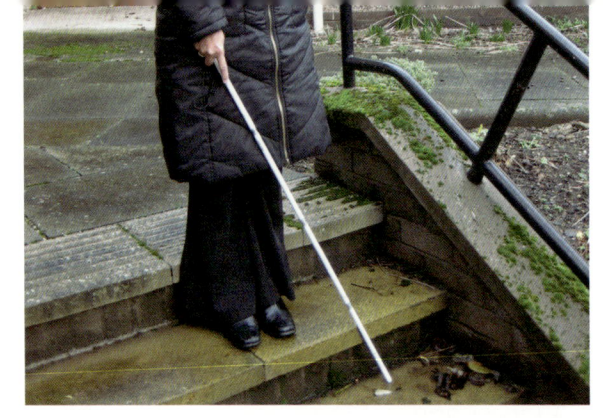

Guide cane.

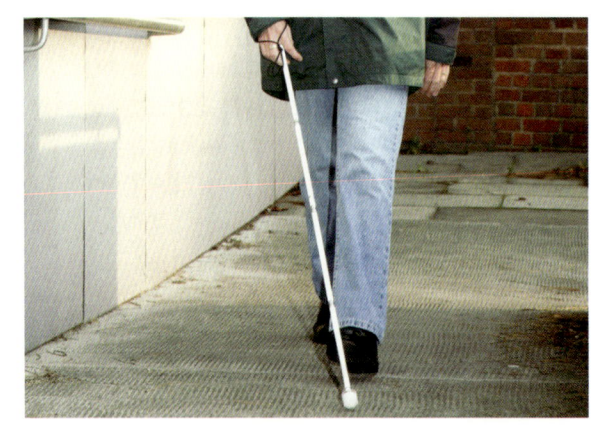

Long cane.

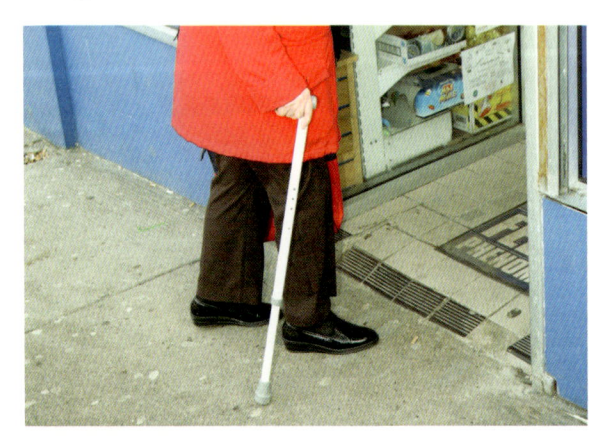

Walking stick.

- People using red and white striped canes have both visual and hearing impairment.

5. Electronic Visual Enhancement Systems (EVES)[6]

Sonic aids use projected sound waves to determine the presence and distance of nearby objects (similar to radar).

Global Positioning Systems (GPS) are similar to those used in car navigation, and can inform the user of their specific location to a matter of metres, assisting with location-specific warnings and information.

6. Making things bigger

Large print can allow a more natural reading position, needs no training to use and has less stigma attached than magnifiers. Physical constraints such as size and weight limit the range of magnification. The size of commercially produced large print varies from 14 to 24 point (Figure 5).

Ophthalmology services should provide appointment details and information to patients in at least 14 point print. Patients and their friends and families

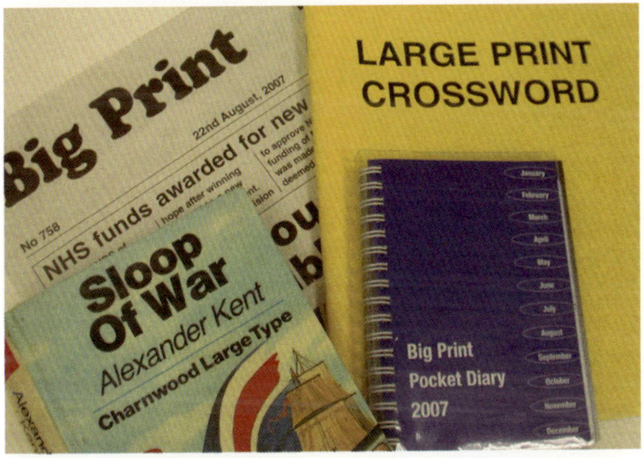

Figure 5: Various large print materials are available, including newspapers, recipe books, puzzle books, calendars, address books, magazines and dictionaries.

should also be encouraged to produce their own large print. Copies of recipes, music and other shorter pieces of text can be made larger using the enlargement facility on photocopiers, although care should be taken because contrast may be reduced. Black felt-tip pens can be used to write large print phone numbers, lists, labels or letters. Computer settings can be adapted to make them easier to use, and good quality large print texts can then be printed.

Many other 'bigger' items are available from social services and local and national voluntary organisations (Figure 6).

7. Improving lighting

Appropriate lighting for people with sight loss is particularly important, because they may be functioning at their visual threshold. The use of magnifiers may not be necessary for certain tasks with adequate illumination. Elderly patients in particular are often unaware of the benefits of improved lighting in the home, and may be reluctant to change their living environment. As many low vision patients suffer from discomfort glare, a change in their use of lighting may also improve comfort.

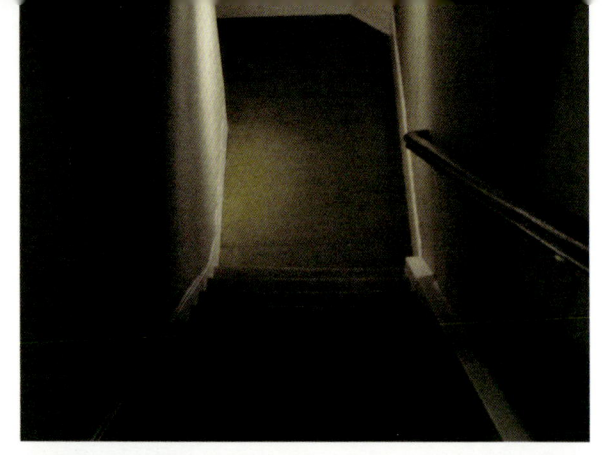

Figure 7: Dimly lit stairs can be dangerous.

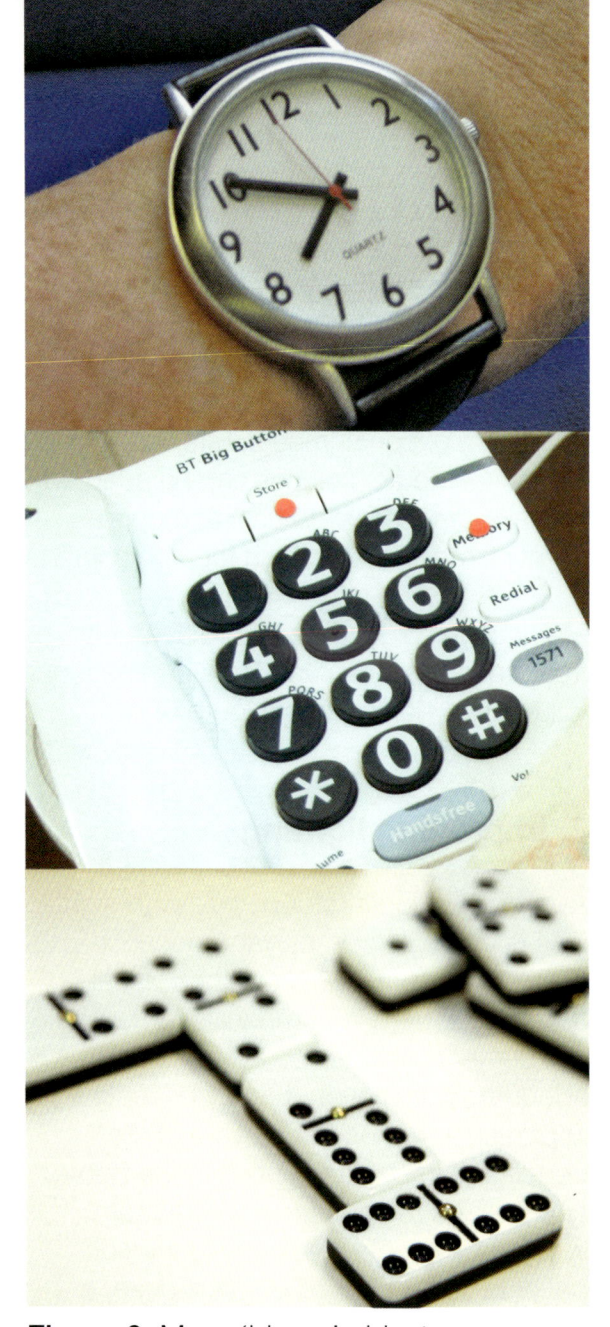

Figure 6: Many 'bigger' objects are available, including watches, telephones and games.

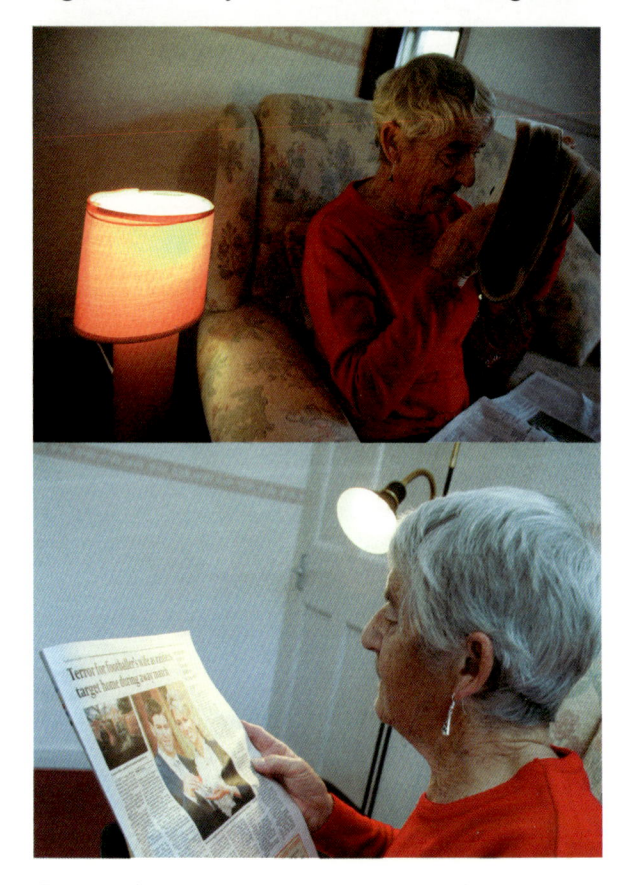

Figure 8: With improved task lighting, a magnifier may not be necessary.

General lighting

This is the lighting used in the home, or other indoor environments, that allows a person to get around and locate objects safely. In the main, people with a visual impairment need greatly increased ambient levels of illuminance. People with poor vision often have longer light-dark adaptation, so it is important to keep light levels throughout the home even. Ceiling spotlights can cause marked differences in light levels and glare problems so are best avoided. Particular attention should be given to stairs and landings by ensuring they are well lit (Figure 7).

Task lighting

Localised task lighting is required for reading, using the telephone, over kitchen work surfaces and above eating areas. Table and standard lamps, which many people have in their homes as task lights, are not useful in a low vision context (Figure 8).

Adjustable angle-poise lamps are best for reading. The best position is below eye level, between the person and what they want to see. Incandescent tungsten lamps (filament bulbs) are very cheap and can be used in task lamps that are not required for prolonged periods, such as a lamp over the telephone. However, if used for a prolonged period they can cause discomfort as they emit heat. Many adjustable task lights are now available with compact fluorescent tubes. These are the bulbs of choice for prolonged reading tasks because they produce an even light and generate very little heat. Although they are more expensive to buy, they last about 10 times as long as standard light bulbs and use less electricity.

8. Reducing glare

Visors and shields

Visors and shields protect from glare sources while not obstructing the rays of light from the object being viewed. Patients may wear sports peaks or a hat with a brim. Side shields are also useful if permanently attached to spectacles.

Tints

Prescribing tints for people with low vision is not easy. Many patients ask for a dark tint because they find bright lights outside distressing. However, the same people often need more light for near tasks and getting about safely. For a small number of patients who are photophobic (for instance, with albinism), the constant wear of tints may be necessary. However, for the vast majority of low vision patients flexibility is required. For most, the best solution is a cheap plano sunspec or overspec that has side and top shields and can be removed or put on quickly (Figure 9).

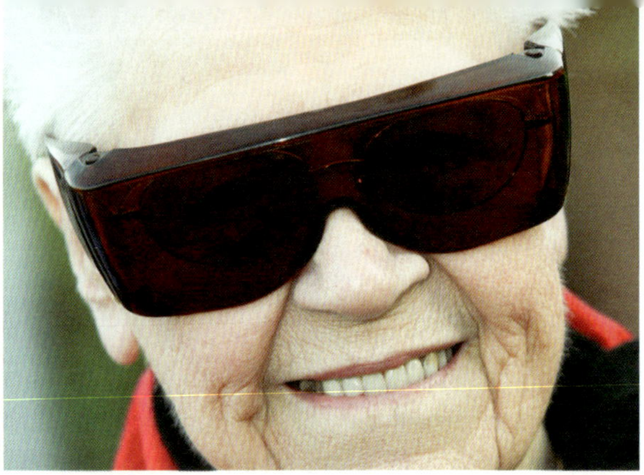

Tints for glare

Discomfort glare can be removed by reducing light with a tint. The patient should be given the opportunity to choose the depth of a neutral density tint they like best – it may be helpful if they try different tints while walking around outside.

To reduce disability glare, and hence improve the retinal image contrast, a tint needs to absorb the light scattered in the eye, whilst ensuring un-scattered light is not reduced. A grey neutral density filter will simply reduce all the light and hence not change the contrast of the retinal image.

Blue light is scattered more than red light by the lens, and is also thought to be more harmful to the macula. Therefore, yellow, amber and brown tints, which absorb shorter wavelengths of light, have been suggested as being of benefit to patients with low vision who suffer from disability glare. Results of research into the success of these tints in improving visual performance in low vision patients is mixed: Bailey et al[7] found that they reduced reading performance; Wolffsohn et al[8] showed that yellow and orange tints

Figure 9: Tinted overshields.

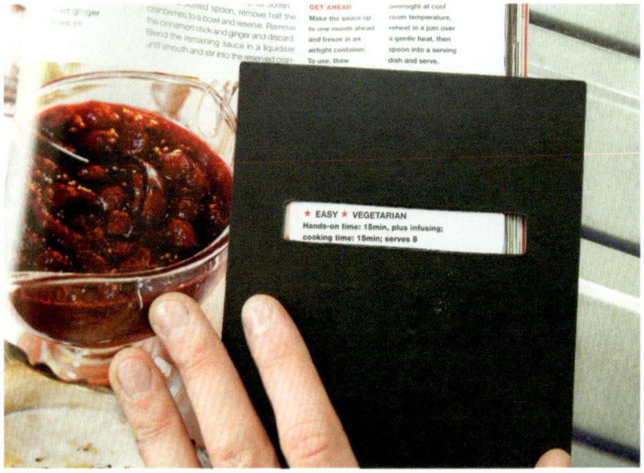

Figure 10: A typoscope.

increased contrast sensitivity in people with AMD.

Dark red tints, which do not transmit any light less than 550nm, have traditionally been prescribed for people with retinitis pigmentosa and albinism. There is no evidence of their success over and above equivalent neutral density filters.

Typoscopes

A typoscope is a rectangular black card with a central slit (Figure 10). In some cases reflected light on a page acts as a glare source, and is scattered in the eye thus reducing the contrast of the retinal image. This is particularly apparent in patients with media opacities. A typoscope reduces the amount of light from the background, reduces scatter and thus increases the retinal image contrast.

9. Improving contrast

Low vision patients have poor sensitivity to low contrast targets. There are many ways a person can improve contrast in their daily lives. Some examples are:

- Using Closed Circuit Televisions (CCTVs), which enhance the luminance contrast and can reverse contrast (i.e. white print on a black background).
- Writing with a black felt-tip pen on white paper, which produces higher contrast letters.
- Putting white strips on the edge of darkly coloured stairs.
- Painting walls, floors, ceilings, doors and doorframes contrasting colours to make them easier to see.
- Chopping vegetables on contrasting chopping boards, e.g. an onion on a red board and a tomato on a white board.
- Marking switches and dials with contrasting coloured bump-ons.

10. Environmental adaptations

A detailed discussion of environmental adaptations is available in specialised texts[3,9]. Since the introduction of the Disability Discrimination Act[10], there has been a dramatic improvement in adaptations to public places for people with a visual impairment, including talking, large print and Braille signs, tactile pavements and contrasting colour schemes. Under the same Act, providers of health services are required to make reasonable adjustments to their practices to make them accessible to people with a disability, including people with a visual impairment.

11. Sight substitution

Over 80 per cent of information from the world around us comes from the sense of sight. Even when sight is impaired, it may still be the prominent sense. Other senses, mainly hearing and touch, may be used for some tasks but many people choose to use a mixture of sight substitution methods and sight enhancement. For example, a person may choose to read a newspaper or magazine using a magnifier, but find talking books easier for longer novels. It is untrue that people with a visual impairment have an enhanced sense of hearing and touch – they have simply had more practice using them.

Many items are available which use sound and texture to assist people with a visual impairment with daily living tasks (Figure 11). These include:
- A liquid level indicator, which beeps when the liquid reaches it, so that cups or jugs are not over-filled.
- Audio-described videos and DVDs, which are now available in many popular titles. The story is narrated over the original film.
- Talking microwaves, clocks, watches, thermometers and scales.
- Games with tactile counters, boards and cards.
- Bump-ons which can be used to mark dials on appliances so that positions can be seen and felt.

Braille and Moon
Braille is the best-known method of tactile reading and writing. Particular combinations of up to six raised dots,

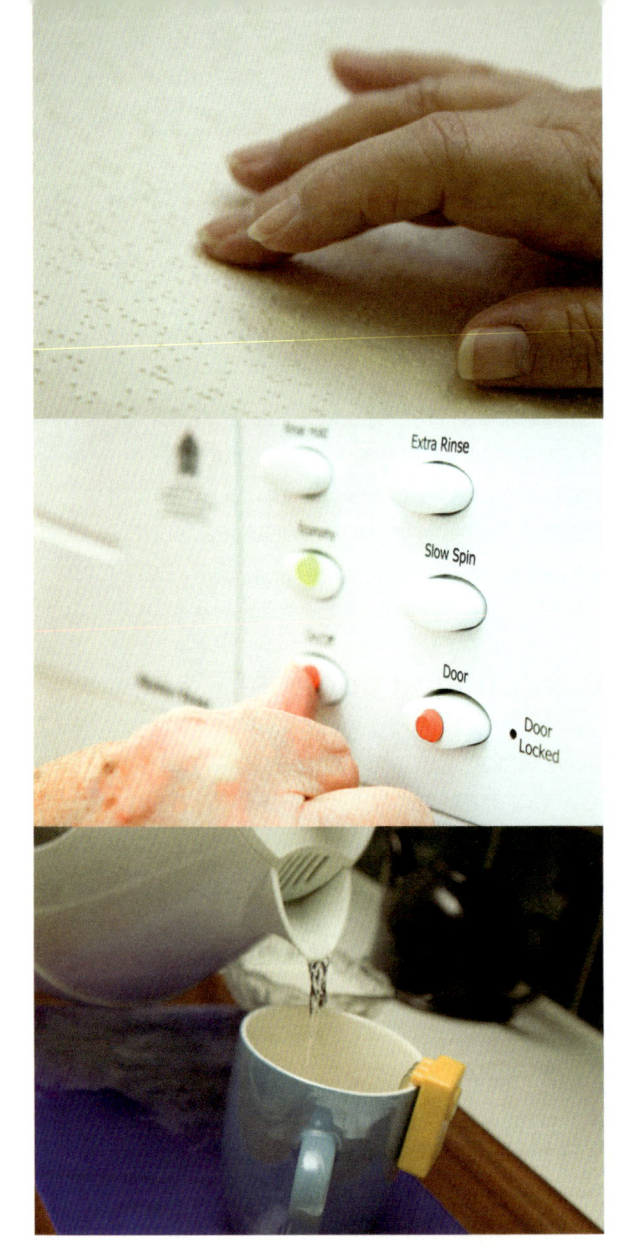

Figure 11: Many items are available which use sound and texture to assist people with a visual impairment, including Braille, bump-ons to mark up dials, and a liquid level indicator.

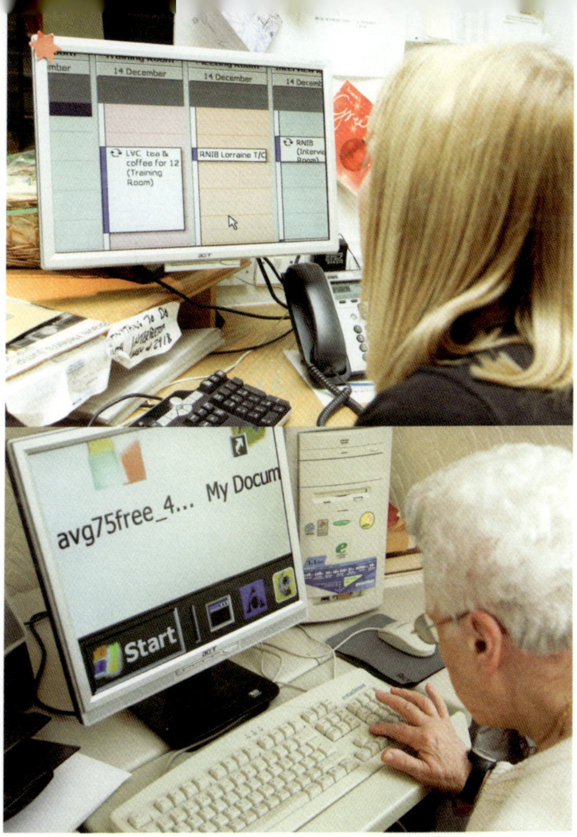

Figure 12: Computer adaptations for people with a visual impairment have progressed rapidly.

arranged like the numbers on a dice, produce each of the 63 symbols. Relatively few people read and write Braille; less than 10 per cent of blind people in the UK can write it. People may use it for labelling and for short texts rather than for reading books. Most Braille users are congenitally blind, and will have learned it at school. However, most rehabilitation workers can teach it to adults.

Moon is simpler to learn than Braille since its shape resembles letters, but very few people use it and there are not many books available in this format.

Talking books, newspapers and magazines

The RNIB's talking book service currently holds over 13,000 titles which can be played on user-friendly machines. For an annual subscription, often paid by the Local Authority, an unlimited number of titles can be sent out and returned free of postage charge.

The Talking Newspaper Association of the UK is a national charity co-ordinating voluntary groups who produce versions of their local newspaper on tape, CD and email. The central organisation produces versions of national newspapers and magazines, of which there are currently about 400 titles. For a fixed annual fee a person can receive as many of these as they wish.

12. Computers and visual impairment

As with all computer technology, adaptations for people with a visual impairment have progressed rapidly in recent years. Both sight enhancement and sensory substitution techniques can be employed so that anyone with a visual impairment, regardless of their level of vision, can use them (Figure 12).

Navigation around a computer can be aided by magnifying or speech output software, and the contrast and colours can be changed easily. The information in a document can be enlarged, read to the user or processed onto a Braille pad. Input can be via a keypad with large characters or Braille characters, or speech. The equipment exists to allow the image from a CCTV to be displayed on a split screen with the computer document, and printing can be in large print or Braille.

References

1. Nilsson UL, Frennesson C, Nilsson SEG. Patients with AMD and a large absolute central scotoma can be trained successfully to use eccentric viewing, as demonstrated in a scanning laser ophthalmoscope. Vis Res 2003;43(16):1777-1787.
2. Macnaughton J. Low vision assessment. Philadelphia: Elsevier-Butterworth-Heinemann, 2005.
3. Dickinson C. Low Vision Principles and Practice. Oxford: Butterworth-Heinemann, 1998.
4. www.rnib.org.uk. How to guide people with sight problems. London: RNIB.
5. www.guidedogs.org.uk
6. Wolffsohn JS, Peterson RC. Current knowledge on electronic vision enhancement systems (EVES) for the visually-impaired. Ophthal Physiol Optics 2003;23:35-42.
7. Bailey IL, Kelty K, Pittler G, Raasch T, G. R. Typoscopes and yellow filters for cataract patients. Low Vision Abstracts 1978;4:2-6.
8. Wolffsohn JS, Dinardo C, Vingrys AJ. Benefit of coloured lenses for age-related macular degeneration. Ophthal Physiol Optics 2002;22:300-311.
9. Barker P, Barrick J, Wilson R. Building sight. London: RNIB/HMSO, 1995.
10. Disability Discrimination Act. London: HMSO, 1995.

Low vision in children

Introduction

Visual impairment in childhood has implications for the future of the child and the immediate family. As the child's potential in terms of education, employment, emotional development and socialising skills will all be influenced, it is critically important that appropriate support is given to minimise any consequent handicap[1,2]. Low vision services have an important role in visual assessment, provision of aids and making appropriate recommendations in respect of the child's visual environment.

Epidemiology

Serious visual loss in childhood is uncommon, with six of every 10,000 children born in the UK each year becoming blind by their 16th birthday, and probably a further 12 becoming visually-impaired (worse than 6/18)[3].

Thus there are at least four newly visually-impaired children each day in the UK, and two per 1,000 children in a given population at any time are visually-impaired or blind[4].

In developed countries, cerebral visual impairment is the most common cause of poor vision in children. A study of blind certifications in England and Wales from 1999-2000 (Table 1) found that 41.2 per cent of certifications in children were for cerebral visual impairment and disorders of the optic nerve[5]. At least 75 per cent of such children have disorders that are neither potentially treatable nor preventable with current knowledge[3]. The main challenge is therefore in developing services to habilitate these children.

Children with cerebral visual impairment are more likely to have additional disabilities than children in whom visual impairment is due to the eye or optic nerve[4,6]. Less than 10 per cent of visually-impaired children acquire their sight loss after their first month of life[7,8]. However, progressive conditions such as retinitis pigmentosa and Leber's optic atrophy may worsen during childhood.

Cerebral visual impairment and disorders of the optic nerve	41.2%
Hereditary retinal disorders	13.1%
Congenital anomalies of the eye	13.4%
Perinatal conditions including ROP	8.8%

Table 1: Causes of blindness in England and Wales ages 0-15 years: April 1999-March 2000[5]

Breaking news of visual impairment in a child

In the late 1980s, the Royal National Institute of Blind People (RNIB) interviewed a group of parents of visually-impaired children to identify the needs of the parents and children around the time of diagnosis of visual impairment[9]. In the resulting guideline for good practice, 'Taking the Time', the multi-disciplinary study group highlighted the following:

"Parents want ophthalmologists to be warm, caring and show empathy, offer positive goals, give them time to listen, consider their needs and treat them with respect. They want honest information, and where there is uncertainty, an acknowledgement that the consultant may not have all the answers at that time. Once they have been told their child is blind or partially-sighted, parents are likely to be in shock and unlikely to retain much information. For this reason, a follow up appointment within two weeks is recommended. A tape recording of the discussion for the parents to take away may also be helpful. It is also important where appropriate to talk directly to the child in language they will understand, and not only to their parents. For these reasons it is also important to offer written information in accessible non-medical jargon with an appropriate reading age."

Although only 16 per cent had received specialist counselling, almost half of parents surveyed said they would have found it very helpful to have someone to talk to about their feelings. Parents needed information on specialist equipment, welfare benefits, educational options, genetic implications and long term prospects.

Children and their families are likely to have contact with many professionals, which can be very time-consuming, repetitive and confusing. The employment of a key worker within a paediatric ophthalmology department has been shown to have benefits for patients, parents and other professionals within the team[10] and this concept is also endorsed in the Royal College of Ophthalmologists' report on Ophthalmic Services for Children[11].

It is advisable to be cautious about giving a definite visual prognosis to parents of young children who appear to be blind. As it is difficult to predict the final visual outcome in young children, it is important to avoid judging the child's visual function too early in life. Whilst it is essential that parents are not given unrealistic expectations of their child's future vision, it is important to remember that some children with serious ocular disorders and apparently very poor vision can achieve better than expected overall visual ability[12].

Registration of children

When a child is registered as visually-impaired, services and advice become more accessible, especially if the special education department works closely with the local visual impairment society.

A child with a visual impairment may be registered on one or more of the following:

1. **The blind and partial sighted register (as outlined in Chapter 3)**
   The special guidance in relation to children states that: "Infants and young children who have congenital ocular abnormalities leading to visual defects should be certified as sight impaired unless they are obviously severely sight impaired. Children aged four and over should be certified as severely sight impaired or sight impaired according to the binocular corrected vision."

   This system was not devised for the needs of children, and has changed little since its inception. As a consequence, it is inappropriate for children and their educational needs and is not usually used as the main trigger for services.

   In practice, most children with sight loss present to hospital eye services within their first year of life. Screening of high risk neonates (with conditions associated with visual impairment, or for retinopathy of prematurity or periventricular leukomalacia) may detect abnormalities which require further investigation. Referral may also occur in response to parental suspicion of impaired vision.

The consultant paediatric ophthalmologist will decide at what stage to raise the issue of registration, but this is unlikely to be at the first visit. The potential advantages of registration should be discussed with an unhurried approach and concerns about the possible stigma of registration should be allayed. However, it is of the greatest importance that time is not lost in waiting for the registration to be carried out before the child and parents are referred for specialist support services.

2. **Register of children with special educational needs**
Registers are kept by each school and each Education Authority. The register details the help to be provided to the child. Statements of Special Educational Needs (SEN) were introduced following the Education Act 1981[13]. In Scotland, the equivalent strategic support plan is the Record of Needs[14]. Many children with significant visual impairment and who also have a legal statement of special educational needs will fail to meet the criteria for blind or partially-sighted registration.

3. **Register of children with a disability**
The Children Act[15] 1989 imposes a general duty on local councils to provide a range of services to 'children in need' in their area. Social services keep a register of children with a disability in each locality. Inclusion on this list acts as the main trigger for social services provision for children. The purpose of the register is to enable children's services, health and voluntary services to work more closely together to identify and plan for children and young people with a disability and their parents/carers.

Education services

Children with a visual impairment have a right to educational assistance as laid down by the Children Act 1989[15]. The way in which this assistance should be provided is outlined in the Education Act 1993[16], and from this the Department of Education and Skills has derived a code of practice. The code, which was revised in 2001, sets out the procedures that the education system follows in order to identify and assess children with special educational needs, including children with a visual impairment. If the child's progress is causing concern, the class teacher approaches parents to discuss how they might work together to tackle the problem.

1. School action
The school's Special Educational Needs Co-ordinator (SENCO) assesses the child's learning difficulty and produces an Individual Education Plan (IEP). This is monitored and reviewed regularly and may include individual tuition, special adaptations and equipment such as low vision aids.

2. School action plus
The school calls upon external specialist support, such as a specialist teacher for the visually-impaired or an educational psychologist, to help formulate a new IEP.

3. Statutory assessment
The Local Education Authority makes a statutory assessment of special educational needs. The needs of the child are assessed by the school, outside professionals and family. A Local Education Authority panel then considers input from a variety of sources:

- Parents
- Qualified teacher for the visually-impaired
- GP, ophthalmologist, optometrist and/or paediatrician
- Educational psychologist
- Social services.

4. A statement of the special educational needs
of the child is agreed by the panel and issued. The statement binds the Local Education Authority to a range of extra teaching and education provision. Where complex needs are identified, for example the need for a CCTV, adapted computer, personal readers or Braille transcription, a statutory assessment is required. The IEP is reviewed every year. At age 14 a transition plan is drawn up for the move to further education or to the workplace.

The above steps in the process are not always followed in chronological order. Most children with a visual impairment will automatically be referred to a specialist teacher for the visually-impaired as a first step, and some may enter the education system with a statement of special educational needs. In many cases the SENCO will co-ordinate the required support in a completely mainstream environment.

Some children attend schools with specialist units, and a very small number may attend specialist schools for children with a visual impairment. Children with low vision may also benefit from input from other professionals, such as orthoptists, orientation and mobility teachers, educational psychologists, occupational therapists and physiotherapists. Prior to the Warnock Report 1978[17], children with visual impairment were largely educated in specialist schools. Since that time, and with subsequent Education Acts, the emphasis has changed so that now children with visual impairment are included in mainstream schools. This has necessitated the adaptation of teaching materials and the use of specialised equipment, including more extensive use of low vision aids.

An estimated 80 per cent of school tasks are based on vision[18]. It is therefore essential that each child is enabled to maximise the use of their residual vision.

Visual assessment

Visual assessment follows the same principles as for adults (see Chapter 2). Different means of assessment are used depending on a child's developmental age, level of vision and ability to cooperate and communicate. A brief description of some relevant tests will be given, but a full discussion of ophthalmic examination of children is beyond the remit of this text.

For very young children, or older children with communication difficulties, the technique of preferential looking is used. The examiner observes the child's eye movements in response to a target placed in one half of an otherwise blank card, e.g. the Cardiff Acuity Test (Figure 1).

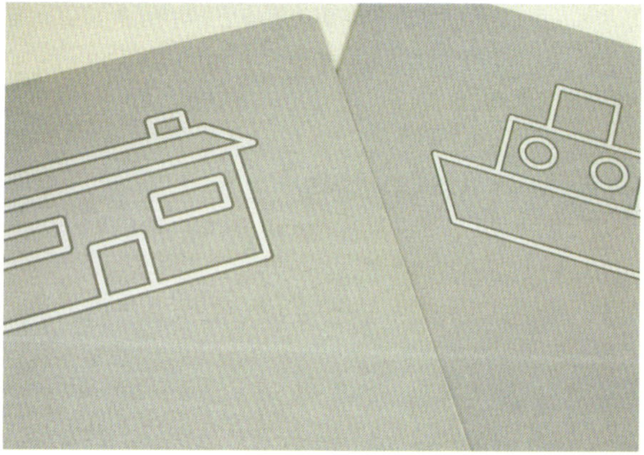

Figure 1: Cardiff Acuity Test.

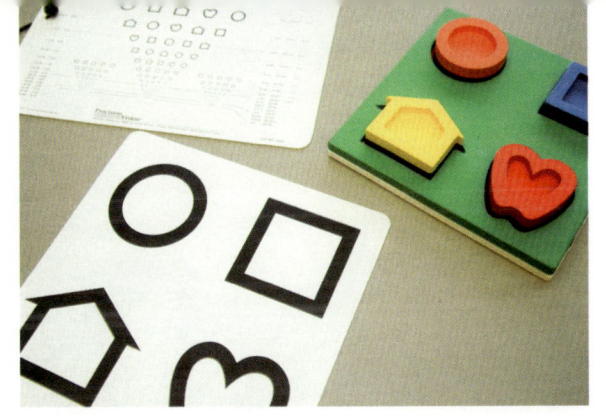

Figure 2: Lea Symbols.

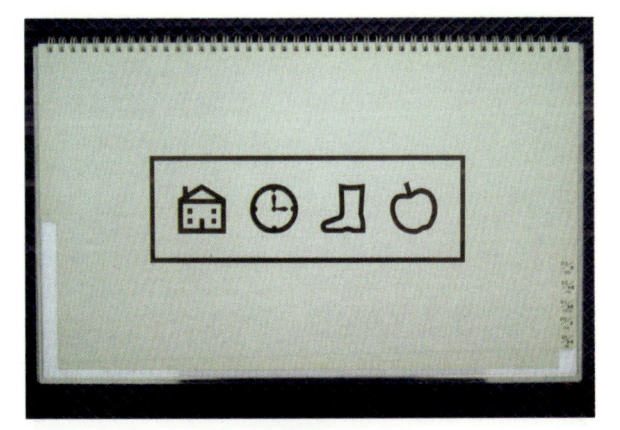

Figure 3: Kay Pictures.

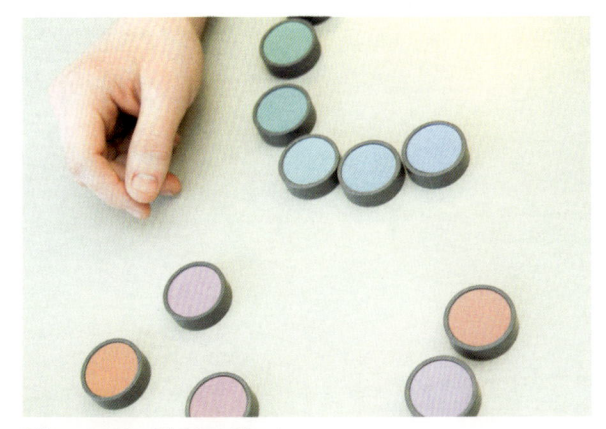

Figure 4: PV16 Test.

For older or more able children, distance visual acuity can be assessed by object recognition and matching e.g. Lea Symbols (Figure 2) or Kay Pictures (Figure 3), both of which allow for logMAR acuity testing by naming, signing or matching symbols.

Conventional near visual acuity is specified by print size. For children who can read, the McClure Reading Test has reading material of varying difficulty appropriate for different ages. For children not yet able to read, acuity is specified for pictures or symbols equivalent to distant targets. The Cardiff Near Test, Kay Pictures Near Test and Lea Symbols Near Test are all suitable, but it is not possible to extrapolate from an acuity value on these tests to a reading print size.

Contrast sensitivity can be tested in younger children by preferential looking with the Cardiff Contrast Test when Pelli-Robson is too difficult. By sequentially presenting increasingly paler faces and observing the child's response, an idea of the child's ability to detect subtle shades of grey is gained. The PV16 is useful for assessing colour vision in children (Figure 4).

A report concerning the child's visual function should be written in plain language and distributed to the multi-disciplinary team. In this way, a child can benefit from all professionals being better informed.

Low vision aids (LVAs)

An up to date refraction is a prerequisite for children being assessed for low vision aids. Lennon et al found that 70 per cent of the previously non-spectacle wearers attending a paediatric low vision clinic were found to require a refractive correction[19]. Children can use their accommodation to great advantage to achieve relative distance magnification by holding objects at a closer viewing distance.

The magnifiers most commonly used by children are flat field (paperweight) magnifiers for near work[7,20,21,22]. They are very easy to use but at 1.8x have limited magnification (Figure 5). Hand magnifiers can be useful for having a quick look at something very small, including three-dimensional objects (Figure 6). Distance magnification is best achieved with binoculars (Figure 7), or if the child is older and can hold steady fixation, a more discreet telescope. The magnification

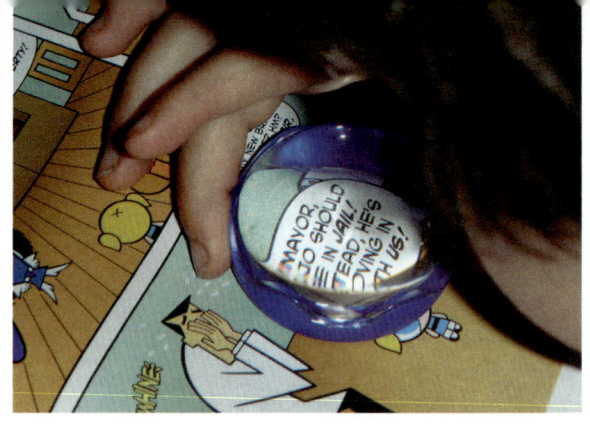

Figure 5: Flat field magnifier.

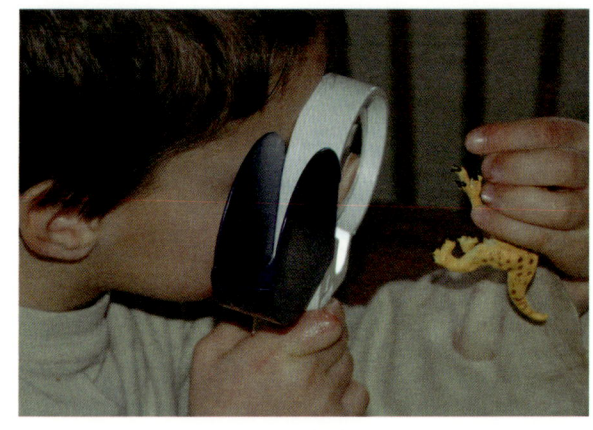

Figure 6: Hand magnifier.

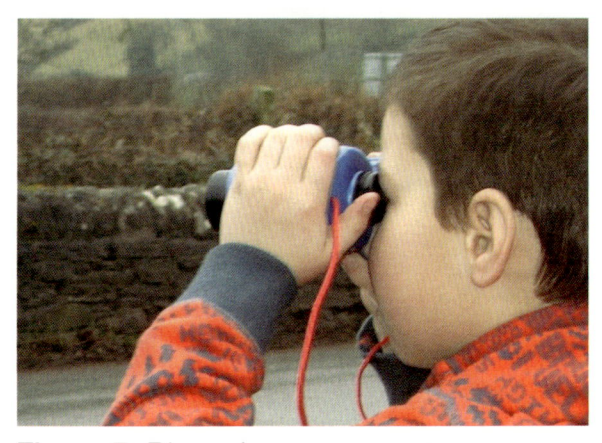

Figure 7: Binoculars.

power of such aids is usually between 4x and 8x magnification. Training is required to use them to quickly search and focus, and good eye-hand coordination is required to track targets.

Non-optical aids are just as useful for children as for adults. Glare can be a problem, especially for children with conditions such as albinism. Tints incorporated into lenses may therefore be helpful. Peaked caps are also useful in this regard, but as with all aids for children, reluctance to stand out from the crowd may limit the use of conspicuous adaptations. Other non-optical aids include reading stands, task lighting, Closed Circuit Television (CCTV) and adapted computers. Early intervention with low vision aids can improve long term visual functioning, and there is evidence that their use should ideally begin before children enter primary education[22,23].

Support services

While education services usually take the leading role in coordinating services for visually-impaired children, each child will have specific needs outside the school setting as well as in the classroom, and these should be addressed by local social services. Rehabilitation workers can teach children orientation and mobility and independent living skills, and help with social communication. A social worker may offer advice on financial benefits to which the family is entitled, and counselling or other emotional support.

References

1. Speedwell L, Stanton F, Nischal KK. Informing parents of visually-impaired children: who should do it and when? Child Care Health Dev. 2003;3:219-24.
2. Youngson-Reilly S, Tobin MJ, Fielder AR. Patterns of professional involvement with parents of visually-impaired children. Developmental Medicine and Child Neurology 1994;36:449-458.
3. Rahi JS, Cable N. Severe visual impairment and blindness in children in the UK. Lancet 2003;362:1359-1365.
4. Rahi J, Dezateux C. Epidemiology of Visual Impairment. In: David T, editor. Recent Advances in Paediatrics. London: Churchill Livingstone, 2001:97-114
5. Bunce C, Wormald R. Causes of blind certifications in England and Wales: April 1999-March 2000. Eye, 2007. (E-published ahead of print)
6. Hou R, Burden SK, Hoyt CS, Good WV. Chronic Cortical Visual Impairment in Children: Aetiology, Prognosis and Associated Neurological Deficits. Br J Ophthalmol 1999;6:670-5.
7. A New System of Notification of Childhood Visual Impairment and the Information it has Provided on Services for Scottish Children Edinburgh. Vision Impairment Scotland, 2003.
8. Blohme J, Tornqvist K. Visual Impairment in Swedish Children. II. Etiological factors. Acta Ophthalmol.Scand 1997;75:199-205.
9. RNIB. Taking the Time: telling parents their child is blind or partially-sighted. London: RNIB, 1998.
10. Rahi JS, Manaras I, Tuomainen H, Hundt GL. Meeting the needs of parents around the time of diagnosis of disability among their children: evaluation of a novel program for information, support, and liaison by key workers. Paediatrics 2004;114:477-82.
11. Clarke M. Ophthalmic Services for Children. London: RCOphth, 2005.
12. Jugnoo S, Rahi J. Examination of a Child with Visual Loss. Community Eye Health 1998;27:36-38.
13. Education Act. London: HMSO 1981.
14. Education (Additional Support for Learning) (Scotland) Bill 2003.
15. The Children Act. London: HMSO 1989.
16. The Education Act. London: HMSO 1993.

References (continued)

17. Warnock Committee. Special Educational Needs: Report of the Enquiry into the Education of Handicapped Children and Young People. London, 1978.
18. Kelley PA, Sanspree MJ, Davidson RC. Vision Impairment in Children and Youth. In: Silverstone B, Lang MA, Rosenthall B, Faye EE, editors. The Lighthouse Handbook on Vision Impairment and Vision Rehabilitation. Oxford University Press, 2000:1137-51.
19. Lennon J, Harper R, Biswas S, Lloyd C. Paediatric low-vision assessment and management in a specialist clinic in the UK. Br J Vis Impair 2007;25:103-119.
20. Ruddock G, Corcoran H, Davies K. Developing an Integrated Paediatric Low Vision Service. Ophthal Physiol Opt 2004;24:323-326.
21. Lee S, Cho J. Low vision devices for children. Community Eye Health 2007;20:28-29.
22. Gould E, Sonksen P. A Low Visual Aid Clinic for Pre-school Children. Br J Vis Impair 1991;9:44-46.
23. Leat SJ. Paediatric Low Vision Management. CE Optom 2002;5:22-5.

Does he have to be so blind?

We've seen a multitude this morning
And there's still one more to see
But at least this one's a quickie –
Just a dry ARMD.

She seems a bright old lady
Hope she doesn't ask too much
A few words of reassurance
And with luck I'll get some lunch.

"Wear and tear" – what does he mean?
And "failing circulation"?
But "no, I never will go blind
I'll keep my navigation".

He's smiling as he says it
And I'm smiling back at him
His voice is smooth and kindly
But his face is blurred and dim.

"If things get worse tell your GP
About the situation
Then we'll arrange to have you back
And do your registration.

"I'm sorry we can do no more
For you, but never fear –
It may not get much worse than this
So chin up now my dear."

Oh let me out, let me out
Before I leave in tears.
Why must he patronise me?
Oh, please let me out of here.

Can't he see I'm numb with horror
While he's trying to be kind?
Can't he see my world just ended…
Does he have to be so blind?

Index

Accessible information	20
Amsler Grid	28
Angular magnification	49
Appointment letters	20
Bad news	28, 64
Bailey-Lovie	26
BD8	14, 34
Binoculars	49, 70
Blind registration	32-34, 66
BP1	33
Braille	60-62
Breaking bad news	28, 64
Bump-ons	59, 60
Cardiff Acuity Cards	68
Cardiff Contrast Test	69
CCTVs	47, 48, 62, 71
Certification benefits	32, 36
criteria	33, 35
England	34
forms	32-34
Northern Ireland	34
process	33-37
Scotland	33
terminology	33-37
Wales	34
Charles Bonnet Syndrome	25
Children	63-73
Closed Circuit Televisions	47, 48, 62, 71
Colour vision	69
Community Care	39, 40
Computer adaptations	61, 62
Contrast	59
Contrast sensitivity	26, 58
Contrasting colours	59
Cooking	23
Counselling	30, 40, 64, 71
CVI	34
Daily living skills	40
Dark adaptation	25
Disability Discrimination Act	59
Distance low vision aids	49, 70
Dual sensory loss	24
Eccentric fixation	52
Eccentric viewing	51
Education	66-68
Education Act	66
Electronic Visual Enhancement Systems (EVES)	54
Employment services	41-42
Environmental adaptations	59
Equipment	62, 64, 67-68
Eye Clinic Liaison Officer (ECLO)	22
Falls/falling	23, 27
Families	22, 55, 65
Field expanders	52
Field of view	45, 46

Flat field magnifiers	49, 70
Glare	24, 57-58
Global Positioning Systems (GPS)	54
Guide cane	53, 54
Guide dogs	52, 53
Guiding	21-22, 52
Hallucinations	25
Hand magnifiers	46, 70
Head mounted CCTVs	48
Hearing impairment	24, 39
History taking	22
Individual Education Plan (IEP)	67
Kay Pictures	69
Large print	44, 54-55
Lea Symbols	69
Light adaptation	25
Lighting general	25, 55-57
Lighting task	56-57, 71
LogMAR	24-26, 69
Long cane	53, 54
Low vision aids	44-62, 70-71
causes	13-18
definition	12
numbers	13
services	12, 38, 63, 71
therapy	49
LVL	34
Magnification	44-50, 54
Magnification software	62
Magnifiers	44-50, 70-71
McClure Test	69
Medication	24
Minifiers	52
Mirror spectacles	52
Mobility	23, 40, 52-54
Mobility aids	52-54
Moon	60, 61
Orientation and mobility training	23, 40
Overshields	58
Parents	64-65
Partially-sighted registration	14, 32-36
Pelli-Robson	26, 69
Plus lens magnifiers	45-46
Postural aids	51
Prismatic spectacles	52
Psychological support	29-30, 39, 64, 71
PV16	69
Reading books	22, 52-53, 61
computer	48-49
instructions	44
stands	40, 51, 71
Real image magnification	47-49
Refraction	70
Register of children with a disability	66
Register of children with Special Educational Needs	66
Registration benefits	36
criteria	35
England	34
forms	32-35
Northern Ireland	34
process	32-37
Scotland	33
terminology	32-35
Wales	34
Rehabilitation worker	39, 71

Relative distance magnification	44
RVI	34-35
School	67-68
Severely sight impaired	35-36, 65
Shields	57
Sight impaired	35-36, 65
Sight substitution	59-62
Signage	20, 59
Snellen	24, 25
Social services	39-41
Social worker	39, 71
Sonic aids	54
Special Educational Needs Co-ordinator (SENCO)	67
Specialist teachers	67-68
Spectacle mounted magnifiers	46-47
Stand magnifiers	46
Statement of Special Educational Needs	67
Steady eye strategy	52
Symbol cane	53
Talking books	61
Talking magazines	61
Talking newspapers	61
Telephone	23, 36, 56
Telescopes	49, 50, 70
Tints	57-58, 71
Typoscopes	58, 59
Visors	57
Visual acuity	12, 25, 26, 33, 35, 68-69
Visual fields	27-28, 33, 35, 52
Voluntary organisations	42
Warnock Report	68
White sticks and canes	53-54
Working distance	46
World Health Organisation	12, 32